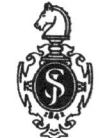

Michael Sticherling
Enno Christophers (eds.)

Treatment of Autoimmune Disorders

With a Foreword
by Karl M. Richter

Springer-Verlag Wien GmbH

Dr. Michael Sticherling
Klinik und Poliklinik für Hautkrankheiten
Universitätsklinikum Leipzig
Leipzig, Federal Republic of Germany

Dr. Dr. h.c. Enno Christophers
Klinik für Dermatologie, Venerologie und Allergologie
Universitätsklinikum Kiel
Kiel, Federal Republic of Germany

Printing was supported by the German Society of Autoimmune Diseases, e.V.

Typesetting: Integra Software Services Pvt. Ltd, Pondicherry
Printed on acid-free and chlorine-free bleached paper
SPIN 10860559

With 32 Figures

ISBN 978-3-211-83772-6   ISBN 978-3-7091-6016-9 (eBook)
DOI 10.1007/978-3-7091-6016-9

Foreword

Under normal circumstances, our immune system is able to distinguish between friend and foe and does not attack the body's own tissues. Unfortunately, this is not always the case. Sometimes the immune system reacts to harmless substances like plant pollen and thus triggers allergic reactions. More serious, however, are autoimmune reactions, which destroy the body's own tissue. Autoimmune disorders may in principal affect any human organ. They therefore have many different clinical faces. Depending on where this attack occurs in the body, different diseases appear. Some antigens and tissues, however, are more frequently involved than others: with regard to multiple sclerosis this is myelin basic protein among different other central nervous system components, in rheumatoid arthritis the innerjoint lining and in diabetes mellitus the insulin-producing cells of the pancreas. In systemic lupus erythematosus, skin, kidneys and various other organs are targeted.

These are only examples. In fact, currently there are more than 60 different autoimmune disorders known and 5% of all adults in Europe and North America suffer from one or more autoimmune disorders. Despite these facts, autoimmune disorders do not attract ample attention neither in the public nor in scientific research. In particular, scientifically based clinical trials on autoimmune disorders are relatively underrepresented because of missing financial support. In addition, autoimmune disorders occur in many different medical specialities which have little communication with each other at both national and international level. Despite similarities of underlying causes and mechanisms, each medical speciality has developed its own treatment principles without taking much notice of progress made in other areas. As a consequence, the German Society of Autoimmune Diseases, e.V. (formerly, Association for Promoting the Treatment of Autoimmune Diseases) is aiming at these deficits and has set its objectives to help to improve this situation.

The main target is to collect clinical and scientific knowledge on autoimmune diseases, the causes which trigger nontolerance and on genetic background, among others. Projects with novel promising therapies should be supported and accelerated through interdisciplinary exchange and cooperation.

This includes mental and financial support by the Society of relevant therapeutic research: distribution of new scientific knowledge, rewarding outstanding scientific studies and organizing international interdisciplinary symposia and conferences.

We hope that among the different activities of the Society this compendium will contribute to help the reader to look over the fence of his or her own medical speciality in order to learn from experiences in the other areas.

> K. M. Richter
> Chairman of the Executive Board
> Association for Promoting the Treatment
> of Autoimmune Diseases

Preface

The human body is constantly exposed to intrinsic and extrinsic factors which threaten the integrity of the organism. In view of the body's constant exposure, it is surprising that diseases do not occur more often. Apparently, efficient protective mechanisms do exist to counteract these attacks. Apart from neoplastic and dys-regulatory disorders, inflammation represents a major part of human pathology. Inflammatory diseases cause a major burden apart from the considerable indivi-dual distress with ensuing disabilities and partly fatal outcome they go along with.

The rapid progress in modern basic and clinical immunology has provided profound knowledge on protective mechanisms against harmful agents from both outside and inside which alter the precisely regulated processes. On the basis of immunosuppressive and immunomodulatory approaches within transplantation medicine, treatment modalities have become available for autoimmune disorders which could so far not be tackled efficiently.

Together with progress in understanding, our attitude towards immunologically related human diseases has profoundly changed. Diseases well-known for a long time have now been recognized as autoimmune mediated. At the same time, established autoimmune diseases can be more conclusively explained.

As a consequence, the concept of autoimmunity is beginning to be appreciated outside the immunological community and both scientific and public awareness of immunologically related disease groups have increased within the last decade. Still many details of the pathogenesis as well as differential therapeutic approaches are unknown among both patients and doctors. Furthermore, scientific exchange across the borders of organ specialization is often limited, though badly needed to improve treatment modalities. Many autoimmune diseases per se as well as long-term treatment periods often result in multiorgan symptoms and call for an interdisciplinary approach.

This is the point where the German Society of Autoimmune Diseases focuses its activities by organizing an annual scientific symposium on interdisciplinary basic and therapeutic aspects of autoimmunity. As a result of such activity, this book is intended to compile the data from different medical specialties and to present and discuss results across the borders of the organs studied within their research. Thus, new ideas and concepts for therapy should be made available to a scientific and clinical community by bringing together basic aspects of auto-immune disorders, current concepts of their treatment as well as experimental and future approaches which will still have to prove their effectiveness. Autoimmune diseases are a subject of basic and clinical research which is in constant change and progress. We sincerely hope to have added a glimpse of the subject by bringing together renown authors within their fields to cover several different human organs which can be affected by autoimmune diseases. Future progress within the field will result in better patient care and symptom relief as the major intention of medical research.

M. Sticherling, E. Christophers

Contents

Definitive T cell epitope mapping for a human disease: gluten challenge in coeliac disease identifies a dominant transglutaminase-deamidated T cell epitope

Robert P. Anderson*

Nuffield Department of Medicine, University of Oxford, John Radcliffe Hospital,
Oxford, United Kingdom

Introduction

Antigen-specific immunotherapy has been proven to be an effective means of preventing and treating antigen-driven immune disease in experimental animals. Human diseases with strong human lymphocyte antigen (HLA) associations such as multiple sclerosis, rheumatoid arthritis and juvenile diabetes are believed to be driven by autoantigens and/or environmental antigens that mimic autoantigens. However, human diseases are generally not amenable to study until clinically manifest, when the pathologic immune response is chronic. In animal models, autoimmune disease can be triggered by immunization with a single peptide derived from a critical autoantigen. This peptide corresponds to a dominant T cell epitope. However, as disease progresses, the immune response diversifies and multiple peptide epitopes derived from the original autoantigen, as well as other proteins in the target tissue, are recognized by cognate T cells. This process is termed epitope spreading and has prevented definitive identification of T cell epitopes and antigens that initiate human disease.

Currently, there is no agreed optimal method for the identification of pathogenic T cell epitopes in human disease. Epitopes have been defined for T cell clones and lines and for fresh T cells from blood or affected tissue or, more recently, by using laboratory animals transgenic for disease-associated human major histocompatibility complex molecules. However, the relevance of such epitopes to disease initiation or maintenance, their importance as dominant or subdominant epitopes and their potential utility as antigen-specific therapeutics are not clear.

* Author's present address: Autoimmunity and Transplantation Division, Walter and Eliza Hall Institute, Parkville, Victoria 3050, Australia.
E-mail: banderson@wehi.edu.au

Our recent studies in coeliac disease contrast with previous "static" T cell epitope mapping relying upon T cell clones and lines. Utilization of antigen (dietary wheat gluten) challenge in vivo in coeliac subjects following a gluten-free diet has allowed T cell epitope mapping to proceed during the early phase of disease reactivation. These studies show a single dominant T cell epitope exists in a model gluten protein, recognized by T cells induced in peripheral blood following gluten challenge. The dominant epitope corresponds to a transglutaminase(tTG)-deamidated 17mer peptide. T cell epitope spreading is found in peripheral blood as early as ten days after gluten challenge. Because antigen exposure is readily manipulated and symptoms associated with disease reactivation are generally mild and rapidly reversible, coeliac disease is unique among human immune-mediated diseases for the dissection of T cell epitope hierarchies and rational development of peptide-based antigen-specific therapies.

HLA-DQ, gluten and coeliac disease

Gluten and HLA-DQ2 are definitively implicated in the aetiopathogenesis of coeliac disease (see review by Sollid 2000). Over 90% of coeliacs possess HLA-DQ2 (encoded by *HLA-DQA1*05* and *HLA-DQB1*02*), and nearly all others are HLA-DQ8. Since HLA-DQ2 and -DQ8 present peptides to CD4 T cells, there has been intense interest in defining the specificity and phenotype of gluten-specific, HLA-DQ-restricted CD4 T cells in coeliac disease.

In coeliac disease, CD4 T cells predominantly secreting Th1-like cytokines appear in the small intestinal lamina propria within hours of gluten challenge in subjects on gluten-free diet. Initial damage to the intestine following gluten challenge in treated coeliac disease is likely to be due to cytokines (for example, gamma interferon [IFN-γ] and tumour necrosis factor [TNF]) secreted by CD4 T cells that activate macrophages causing release of inflammatory mediators and other cytokines that activate other cell types (Nilsen et al. 1998).

Disease chronicity and epitope spreading: relevance to coeliac disease

Experimental autoimmune diseases, such as experimental allergic encephalitis (EAE), can be initiated by immunization of susceptible mice with adjuvant together with myelin basic protein (MBP) or a specific peptide derived from this protein. This peptide corresponds to the "dominant" T cell epitope of MBP (Tuohy et al. 1999). Exactly what the qualities are, in addition to affinity for HLA and resistance to proteolysis during processing, that lead to one peptide in an antigenic protein being dominant are not fully understood (see review by Yewdell and Bennink 1999). As EAE progresses, a variety of other peptides (subdominant epitopes) derived from MBP and other myelin-associated proteins are recognized by specific T cells in a process termed epitope spreading, also seen in human multiple sclerosis (Tuohy et al. 1999).

Interestingly, when MBP-specific T cells are transferred to a healthy recipient, they are initially abundant in spleen and blood. But just before the onset of EAE, MBP-specific T cells disappear from spleen and blood and become abundant at the site of antigen (central nervous system) (Flugel et al. 2001). Consistent with this, oral administration of antigen is initially followed by proliferation of antigen-specific T cells in gut-associated as well as systemic lymphoid tissue (Gutgemann et al. 1998). Furthermore, T cells with identical specificity are found in murine gut epithelium, lamina propria, and the thoracic duct (Arstila et al. 2000).

Taken together, these studies in mice indicate that T cells specific for dominant or subdominant epitopes appear at different time points and may be located in different anatomical sites according to the chronicity of the immune response. And contrary to the widely held view in coeliac disease research (Molberg et al. 1998), T cells with identical specificities are present in gut and extraintestinal sites such as blood in the early phase of immune responses caused by gut antigen.

Multiple toxic peptides in coeliac disease identified by multiple methodologies

In coeliac disease, a variety of in vivo, ex vivo, and in vitro methods have been exploited to search for "toxic" gluten peptides (Weiser et al. 1995, Sollid 2000). A-gliadin, the first fully sequenced wheat gliadin protein (Kasarda et al. 1984), has been used as the archetypal "toxic gluten" protein source for most of these peptides (see Fig. 1). More recently, recombinant gliadins and peptides corresponding to parts of cDNA-derived gliadin sequences have been studied (Arentz-Hansen et al. 2000). In view of the diversity of model systems, some with no relationship to coeliac disease (for example, fetal intestinal explants), it is not surprising that a variety of different peptides have been defined as toxic. In other studies, nonspecific markers of toxicity (for example, epithelial cell height) have been used as surrogates for immunological toxicity. If the primary hypothesis is that coeliac disease is a T-cell-mediated disease, rational identification of "toxic" gluten peptides in coeliac disease should ideally begin with assays designed to detect HLA-DQ2-restricted CD4 T cells that secrete Th1-associated cytokines (for example, IFN-γ).

```
A   1. VRVPVPQLQP QNPSQQQPQE QVPLVQQQQF PGQQQQFPPQ QPYPQPQPFP SQQPYLQLQP
B                                                P

A  61. PQ     PQLPYPQ PQSFPPQQPY PQPQPQYSQP QQPISQQQAQ QQQQQQQQQQ
B         [..]        P R                      Q              Q[..]

A111. QQQILQQILQ QQLIPCMDVV LQQHNIAHAR SQVLQQSTYQ LLQELCCQHL WQIPEQSQCQ
B                    R            GS                Q        Q

A171. AIHNVVHAII LHQQQ   KQQQQ     PSSQVSFQQP LQQYPLGQGS FRPSQQNPQA
B                  [..]      [..]            Q          S

A221. QGSVQPQQLP QFEEIRNLAL QTLPAMCNVY IAPYC    TIAPF GIFGTN
B                                     P   [..]
```

Fig. 1. *A* Amino acid sequence of A-gliadin (Kasarda et al. 1984) used to derive overlapping 15mer peptides in gluten challenge studies (Anderson et al. 2000); *B* residues that deviate from the consensus sequence derived by Clustal W from 61 Genbank *Tricitum aetivum* α- and α/β-gliadin cDNAs; [..] indicates polymorphic insertion

Intestinal T cell clones for identification of toxic gluten peptides

More recently, intestinal T cell clones from duodenal biopsies of coeliac patients on gluten-free diet pulsed with protease-digested gliadin have been used to search for gliadin-specific T cell epitopes (Sjostrom et al. 1998, van der Wal et al. 1999, Arentz-Hansen et al. 2000). These studies have revealed that intestinal T cell clones raised from gliadin-pulsed coeliac intestinal biopsies predominantly recognize deamidated gliadin epitopes (Molberg et al. 1998). T cell epitopes generally correspond to gliadin peptides deamidated by tTG. tTG is induced with inflammation and apoptosis and irreversibly cross-links proteins and peptides via Glu-Lys isopeptide bonds or directly deamidates glutamine residues to glutamate (Aeschilmann and Paulsson 1994). Intestinal tissue, particularly if inflamed, is rich in tTG. Introduction of glutamate in gliadin T cell epitopes by tTG greatly enhances their binding to HLA-DQ2 (Molberg et al. 1998, Arentz-Hansen et al. 2000).

T cell epitope mapping in immune-mediated diseases

In human immune-mediated diseases, T cell epitopes have been mapped with synthetic 15- to 20mers overlapping by 10 residues spanning known antigenic proteins in assays of peripheral blood T cells. In coeliac disease, it has been contended that gliadin-specific peripheral blood T cells are qualitatively different from intestinal T cells (Sollid 2000). Gliadin-specific intestinal T cell clones are generally HLA-DQ2 restricted, while peripheral blood T cell clones are HLA-DR, -DQ, or -DP restricted (Gjersten et al. 1994). However, these studies were performed before the realization that deamidation of gliadin was important for T cell recognition. Hence, contemporary understanding of toxic gluten peptides in the context of coeliac disease as an HLA-DQ2-associated CD4 T-cell-mediated disease has relied upon the identification of epitopes of intestinal T cell clones with protease-digested gliadin with or without deamidation by tTG.

Unfortunately, it is impossible to know whether epitopes of T cell clones are dominant or subdominant, or whether a clone is specific for only a part of a polyclonal T cell response in vivo. Furthermore, recent studies to identify epitopes of gliadin T cell clones have utilized chymotrypsin-digested gliadins (Arentz-Hansen et al. 2000), even though chymotrypsin selectively cleaves peptide bonds following bulky hydrophobic amino acids – the same amino acids known to be anchor residues at the N- and C-terminal end of the HLA-DQ2 binding motif (see review by Sollid 2000), raising the possibility that bioactive peptides may be artefactually truncated or destroyed.

Hence, a variety of data support the hypothesis that coeliac disease could be initiated by a Th1-like HLA-DQ2-restricted CD4 T cell response focused on particular (probably deamidated) gluten peptide(s). However, current methods relying upon T cell clones or challenge of coeliac tissue in vivo or ex vivo are incapable of defining whether peptides are dominant or subdominant in the immunopathogenesis of coeliac disease.

In vivo gluten challenge and peripheral blood epitope mapping to define T cell epitope hierarchies

Antigen challenge of sensitized subjects results in activation of cognate memory T cells. Memory T cells tend to reside at anatomical sites where their cognate antigen was previously encountered. Recently, memory T cells have been divided into "effector" (cytokine-secreting, CCR7[-]) and lymph node-homing subtypes (CCR7[+]) (Sallusto et al. 2000). We reasoned that gluten challenge in healthy HLA-DQ2[+] coeliac subjects following a strict gluten-free diet would reactivate gluten-specific memory T cells. The initial intestinal inflammation documented by others may be driven by effector memory T cells, but the subsequent appearance of T cells in peripheral blood, perhaps homing back to the gut, may reflect the proliferation of gluten-specific T cells in lymphoid tissue during the days after antigen exposure. Hence, the kinetics and frequency of epitope-specific peripheral blood T cells might reveal dominant versus subdominant gluten epitopes.

Synthetic 15mer peptides overlapping by 10 amino acids corresponding to the composite amino acid sequence (rather than cDNA-derived sequence) of A-gliadin (see Fig. 1) with or without in vitro deamidation by tTG were studied in overnight ex vivo IFN-γ ELISpot assays utilizing peripheral blood mononuclear cells (PBMC) (Anderson et al. 2000). IFN-γ ELISpot assays define the frequency of cells secreting IFN-γ and are capable of detecting peptide-specific T cell frequencies as low as 5–10 per million PBMC. Blood was collected from HLA-DQ2[+] healthy noncoeliac and coeliac subjects after gluten-free diet for at least 4 weeks, and then in the 12 days after commencing gluten challenge (200 g of white bread daily for 1/2 day [n = 1], 3 days [n = 10], or 10 days [n = 1]).

Short-term gluten challenge was generally well tolerated by coeliac subjects, 11 of 12 subjects were able to consume 200 g of gluten bread for 3 or more days, and two thirds had only mild symptoms. One subject had abdominal cramps and vomited within 3 h after the first 2 slices of bread. All symptoms resolved within 1 to 3 days after ceasing gluten challenge.

Prior to gluten challenge, no A-gliadin peptide elicited responses in the IFN-γ ELISpot. However, in 11 of 12 coeliac subjects but none of 4 healthy control subjects, there was induction of IFN-γ ELISpot responses on days 4 through 8 for one pool of overlapping peptides only when treated with tTG. In all cases, IFN-γ induction was attributed to 2 peptides overlapping by 10 amino acids (A-gliadin 56–75). Amino acid sequencing demonstrated that only one glutamine residue in A-gliadin 56–75 was susceptible to tTG-mediated deamidation (Q65). Truncations of A-gliadin 56–75 treated with tTG indicated that residues 64–68 (PQLPY) were critical for bioactivity, and that the 17mer QLQPFPQPQLPYPQPQS (57–73) was the optimal peptide. The bioactivity of QLQPFPQPELPYPQPQS was identical to tTG-treated QLQPFPQPQLPYPQPQS, demonstrating that the bioactivity of this peptide was dependent upon a single deamidated glutamine residue (QE65). Immunomagnetic bead depletion of PBMC prior to the addition of peptide showed this peptide-specific immune response was due to CD4 T cells expressing the β_7, but not the α^E integrin protein, indicating that A-gliadin 57–73 QE65-specific T cells express the $\alpha_4\beta_7$ integrin associated with homing to the intestinal lamina propria (Anderson et al. 2001a). Preincubation of PBMC from HLA-DQ2-homozygous subjects with antibody specific for HLA-DQ (but not HLA-DR or HLA-DP) blocks A-gliadin 57–73 QE65 responses, indicating HLA-DQ2 restriction.

In one subject, who consumed only 2 slices of bread, IFN-γ-secreting T cells specific for A-gliadin 57–73 QE65 were induced on day 6 and persisted until day 12. In another subject, who consumed 4 slices of bread daily for 10 days, A-gliadin 57–73 QE65-specific T cells were also present on days 6 through 8. IFN-γ secretion was only induced by A-gliadin 57–73 QE65 in subjects who consumed bread for 3 days. However, PBMC collected on day 11 from the subject who consumed bread for 10 days secreted IFN-γ in response to 6 of 10 pools of tTG-treated A-gliadin peptides (one pool included A-gliadin 57–73). Hence, T cell epitope spreading occurs as early as 10 days after commencing antigen challenge. These studies indicated: (1) in A-gliadin, there is a hierarchy of T cell epitopes with only one dominant T cell epitope; (2) T cells specific for the dominant epitope are present in peripheral blood only transiently after gluten challenge in vivo but have predictable kinetics; (3) gluten challenge induces T cells specific for the same dominant A-gliadin epitope in almost all HLA-DQ2 coeliac subjects.

Gliadin-specific intestinal T cell clones are focused on two peptides closely related to A-gliadin 57–73 QE65

Arentz-Hansen et al. (2000) have shown that two peptides from a panel of 11 recombinant α-gliadins are common epitopes for gliadin-specific intestinal T cell clones. T cell lines specific for one or both of these peptides (QLQPFPQPELPY and PQPELPYPQPELPY) were raised from intestinal biopsies of 17 HLA-DQ2[+] coeliac subjects on gluten-free diet. These peptides closely resemble A-gliadin 57–73 QE65 and contain the core sequence PELPY, supporting the concept that intestinal and peripheral blood T cell responses induced by gluten challenge are qualitatively similar. More importantly, if intestinal and peripheral blood T cell responses have the same specificity, it is likely the ex vivo polyclonal peripheral blood T cell response will be more informative than T cell clones or lines for studies of molecular specificity and definition of T cell epitope hierarchies in coeliac disease.

Comparison of HLA-DQ2-restricted epitopes of T cell clones with A-gliadin 57–73 QE65

We have studied all the known HLA-DQ2-restricted gliadin epitopes (see Table 1) in IFN-γ ELISpot assays with PBMC from HLA-DQ2 coeliac subjects on day 6 of gluten challenge (3 days, 200 g of gluten-containing bread daily) (Anderson et al. 2001b). A-gliadin 31–49 and GDB2 do not induce IFN-γ responses above background levels, while A-gliadin 57–68 QE65 is generally 25% and α2 gliadin 62–75 QE65 QE72 60% as bioactive as A-gliadin 57–73 QE65 at optimal concentrations (25 µg/ml). To determine whether T cells specific for α2 gliadin 62–75 QE65 QE72 are part of the polyclonal T cell response to A-gliadin 57–73 QE65, IFN-γ ELISpot responses to α2 gliadin 62–75 QE65 QE72 or A-gliadin

Table 1. HLA-DQ2-restricted epitopes of gliadin-specific intestinal T cell clones

Epitope name	Sequence
A-gliadin 57–68 (QE65)	QLQPFPQPELPY
α2 gliadin 62–75 (QE65 QE72)	PQPELPYPQPELPY
A-gliadin 31–49	LGQQQPFPPQQPYPQPQPF
Gamma gliadin (GDB2)	QQLPQPEQPQQSFPEQERPF

57–73 QE65 (25 μg/ml) alone or mixed together were compared. There was no difference between A-gliadin 57–73 QE65 alone or mixed with α2 gliadin 62–75 QE65 QE72, suggesting that in vivo T cells specific for α2 gliadin 62–75 QE65 QE72 and/or A-gliadin 57–68 QE65 are simply part of the polyclonal T cell response targeting A-gliadin 57–73 QE65.

A-gliadin 57–73 QE65 is the optimal α-, α/β-gliadin polymorphism

A-gliadin 57–73 spans a highly polymorphic region of the α-, α/β-gliadins (see Fig. 2) (Anderson et al. 2001b). We have compared IFN-γ ELISpot responses of all the α-, α/β-gliadin polymorphisms of A-gliadin 57–73 found by SwissProt using the search sequence XXXXXXXPQLPYXXXXX. Amongst these polymorphisms, the bioactivity of QLQPFPQPQLPYPQPQ[P,L] is identical to QLQ PFPQPQLPYPQPQS after deamidation by tTG or substitution of QE65. tTG-deamidated PQLPYPQPQLPYPQPQ[P,L] is generally 80% as bioactive as QLQ PFPQPQLPYPQPQS, but substitution of P69 for serine or leucine reduces the bioactivity by 60%. Other polymorphisms are generally less than 20% as bioactive as A-gliadin 57–73. Hence, tTG-deamidated or QE-substituted at position 9,

```
QLQPFPQ..............................PQLPYPQPQP
QLQPFPQ..............................PQLPYSQPQP
QLQPFPQ..............................PQLPYSQPQQ
QLQPFPQ..............................PQLSYSQPQP
QLQPFPQ..............................PQLPYLQPQP
QLQPFSQ..............................PQLPYSQPQP
QLQPFLQ..............................PQLPYSQPQP
QLQPFLQPQPFP..................PQLPYSQPQP
QLQPFPQPQLPYPQPQLPYPQLPYPQPQP
QLQPFPQPQLPYPQ..............PQLPYPQPQP
QLQPFPQPQPFPPQLPYPQPQLPYPQPQP
QLQPFPR..............................PQLPYPQPQP
QLQPFPQPQPFP..................PQLPYPQPPP
QLQPFPQPQPFL..................PQLPYPQPQS
QLQPFPQPQPFP..................PQLPYPQPQS
QPQPFP..............................PQLPYPQTQP
QPQPFPPQ..............................PQLPYPQTQP
```

Fig. 2. Polymorphisms in the region of A-gliadin 57–73 among the 61 *Tricitum aestivum* α-, α/β-gliadin cDNA-derived protein sequences in Genbank

QLQPFPQPQLPYPQPQ[P,L,S] is the α-, α/β-gliadin polymorphism of A-gliadin 57–73 with optimal bioactivity.

One reason for the selection of QLQPFPQPQLPYPQPQ[L,P,S] and PQLP YPQPQLPYPQPQ[P,L] as potent epitopes may be that these sequences are resistant to proteases. Chymotrypsin and pepsin both cleave peptide bonds after hydrophobic residues. In vitro digestion of these peptides and less potent polymorphisms with tyrosine at position 12 followed by proline, serine, or leucine indicates that proline at position 13 prevents susceptibility to both chymotrypsin and pepsin. Hence, it is possible that the specificity of the T cell response is shaped by the susceptibility of gliadin peptides to proteases in the gut (and presumably in antigen presenting cells).

Immune toxicity of wheat, rye and barley due to peptides cross-reactive with A-gliadin 57–73 or epitope spreading initiated by B cells specific for sequences adjacent to A-gliadin 57–73 QE65?

The data we have gathered using PBMC following in vivo gluten challenge in coeliac disease is consistent with A-gliadin 57–73 deamidated by tTG being the dominant α-, α/β-wheat gliadin T cell epitope. Searches for peptides including the core sequence PQLPY have not revealed other wheat, rye, or barley gluten sequences outside the α-, α/β-gliadins of wheat. One possibility is that epitope spreading initiated by the dominant epitope leads to other epitopes in gluten being recognized. Interestingly, B cell epitopes have been identified that are immediately adjacent or including the C- and N-terminal portions of A-gliadin 57–73 (ten Dam et al. 1998, Osman et al. 2000). The other HLA-DQ2-restricted epitopes, gamma gliadin GDB2 and A-gliadin 31–49 are also adjacent to or include sequences identical to or very similar to the same gliadin B cell epitope (QXQPFP). Hence, B-cell-mediated epitope spreading may be initiated by B cells given "help" by T cells specific for the dominant epitope. Alternatively, wheat, rye, and barley may contain prolamin sequences that are cross-reactive with A-gliadin 57–73 but do not include PQLPY, or there are other unique dominant epitopes.

Fine molecular specificity of A-gliadin 57–73 QE65-specific peripheral blood T cells

Residues in A-gliadin 57–73 QE65 that determine bioactivity were mapped by comparing the bioactivity of A-gliadin 57–73 QE65 variants substituted with lysine at each amino acid (Anderson et al. 2001a). Bioactivity was abolished when lysine was substituted at positions 8–11 (PELP) and was substantially reduced with lysine at positions 4–7 (PFPQ) and 12–13 (YP). Single amino acid-substituted variants of A-gliadin 57–73 QE65 with all naturally occurring amino acids except cysteine at positions 4–13 were synthesized and their bioactivity compared to the parent peptide. Positions 4–7 were highly sensitive to substitution – no more than three amino acids at each position conveyed bioactivity greater than 50% of the parent peptide. Positions 4–7 and 12–13 were less sensitive to substitution, but certain amino acids such as proline, lysine, and arginine tended to abolish bioactivity. The fine molecular specificity of peripheral blood T cells for A-gliadin 57–73 QE65 was similar amongst all of the eight coeliac subjects tested. This shared specificity held for residues predicted to be HLA-DQ2 anchor residues (P4, Q7, E9, L10, and Y12) as well as T cell receptor contact residues (F5, P6, P8, P11, and P13).

Antigen-specific therapy using A-gliadin 57–73 QE65

A-gliadin 57–73 QE65 is clearly "the dominant" or "one of the dominant" gliadin T cell epitopes in HLA-DQ2-associated coeliac disease. Therefore, it is reasonable to consider peptide therapeutics based on A-gliadin 57–73 QE65. Peptide delivered orally or nasally would be simple and easy to formulate. Another possibility is the design of altered peptide ligand antagonists that differ from the parent peptide by one or more residues and subtly alter T cell receptor signaling. Altered-peptide ligand antagonists have the potential to "switch off" or "skew" TH1 to TH2 responses in vitro (see review by Bielekova and Martin 2001). We have shown that at least 5 single amino-acid-substituted variants of A-gliadin 57–73 QE65 with weak agonist properties also significantly reduce IFN-γ ELISpot responses to A-gliadin 57–73 QE65 when incubated in 5-fold excess with A-gliadin 57–73 QE65 (unpubl. obs.). It is likely that multiple substitutions or "cocktails" of altered-peptide ligand antagonists will be required for complete blockade of the polyclonal T cell response to A-gliadin 57–73 QE65.

Conclusions

Gluten challenge in coeliac disease allows gliadin-specific T cell responses to be measured and epitope hierarchies to be defined. This method has significant advantages over T cell clones. One dominant T cell epitope has been defined in A-gliadin and is likely to be the dominant α, α/β-wheat gliadin T cell epitope. Whether there are other distinct dominant T cell epitopes in other classes of gliadin in wheat, rye, and barley, or whether toxicity of these proteins is due to cross-reactivity with A-gliadin 57–73 QE65 is crucial to the design of antigen-specific therapeutics. In either case, gluten challenge and testing the bioactivity of peptides and proteins with PBMC will allow the importance of particular epitopes to be determined. The efficacy of altered-peptide ligand antagonists targeting A-gliadin 57–73 QE65 provides proof of principle that peptide therapeutics may be a practical approach to the treatment of coeliac disease without resort to gluten-free diet.

References

Aeschilmann D, Paulsson M (1994) Transglutaminases: protein cross-linking enzymes in tissues and body fluids. Thromb Haemost 71: 402–415

Anderson RP, Degano P, Godkin AJ, Jewell DP, Hill AVS (2000) In vivo antigen challenge in celiac disease identifies a single transglutaminase-modified peptide as the dominant A-gliadin T-cell eptiope. Nat Med 6: 337–342

Anderson RP, Jewell DP, Hill AVS (2001a) Peripheral blood T cells induced by gluten challenge in coeliac disease target a specific molecular motif and express a gut-homing integrin. Gastroenterology 120: A-684

Anderson RP, Jewell DP, Hill AVS (2001b) Bioactivity of peptides homologous to the coeliac-specific dominant A-gliadin T cell epitope. Gastroenterology 120: A-683

Arentz-Hansen H, Korner R, Molberg O, Quarsten H, Van der Wal Y, Kooy YMC, Lundin KEA, Koning F, Roepstorff P, Sollid LM, McAdam SN (2000) The intestinal T cell response to α-gliadin in adult celiac disease is focused on a single deamidated glutamine targeted by tissue transglutaminase. J Exp Med 191: 603–612

Arstila T, Arstila TP, Calbo S, Selz F, Malassis-Seris M, Vassalli P, Kourilsky P, Guy-Grand D (2000) Identical T cell clones are located within the mouse gut epithelium and lamina propria and circulate in the thoracic duct. J Exp Med 191: 823–834

Bielekova B, Martin R (2001) Antigen-specific immunomodulation via altered peptide ligands. J Mol Med 79: 552–565

Flugel A, Berkowicz T, Ritter T, Labeur M, Jenne DE, Li Z, Ellwart JW, Willem M, Lassman H, Wekerle H (2001) Migratory activity and functional changes of green fluorescent effector cells before and during experimental autoimmune encephalitis. Immunity 14: 547–560

Gjertsen HA, Sollid LM, Ek J, Thorsby E, Lundin KEA (1994) T cells from the peripheral blood of coeliac disease patients recognize gluten antigens when presented by HLA-DR, -DQ, or DP molecules. Scand J Immunol 39: 567–574

Gutgeman I, Fahrer AM, Altman JD, Davis MM, Chien Y-h (1998) Induction of rapid T cell activation and tolerance by systemic presentation of an orally administered antigen. Immunity 8: 667–673

Kasarda DD, Okita TW, Bernardin JE, Baeker PA, Nimmo CC, Lew EJ-L, Dietler MD, Greene FC (1984) Nucleic acid (cDNA) and amino acid sequences of α-type gliadins from wheat (*Tricetum aestivum*). Proc Natl Acad Sci USA 81: 4712–4716

Molberg O, McAdam SN, Korner R, Quarsten H, Kristiansen C, Madsen L, Fugger L, Scott H, Roepstorff P, Lundin KEA, Sjorstrom H, Sollid LM (1998) Tissue transglutaminase selectively modifies gliadin peptides that are recognized by gut-derived T cells in celiac disease. Nat Med 4: 713–717

Nilsen EM, Jahnsen FL, Lundin KEA, Johansen F-E, Fausa O, Sollid LM, Jahnsen J, Scott H, Brandtzaeg P (1998) Gluten induces an intestinal cytokine response strongly dominated by interferon gamma in patients with celiac disease. Gastroenterology 115: 551–563

Osman AA, Gunnel T, Dietl A, Uhlig HH, Amin B, Fleckenstein B, Richter T, Mothes T (2000) B cell epitopes of gliadin. Clin Exp Immunol 121: 248–254

Sallusto F, Lenig D, Forster R, Lipp M, Lanzavecchia A (1999) Two subsets of memory T lymphocytes with distinct homing potentials and effector functions. Nature 401: 708–712

Sjostrom H, Lundin KEA, Molberg O, Korner R, McAdam SN, Anthonsen D, Quarsten H, Noren O, Poepstorff P, Thorsby E, Sollid LM (1998) Identification of a gliadin T-cell epitope in coeliac disease: general importance of gliadin deamidation for intestinal T-cell recognition. Scand J Immunol 48: 111–115

Sollid LM (2000) Molecular basis of coeliac disease. Annu Rev Immunol 18: 53–81

ten Dam M, Van de Wal Y, Mearin ML, Kooy Y, Pena S, Drijfhout JW, Koning F, Van Tol M (1998) Anti-alpha-gliadin antibodies (AGA) in the serum of coeliac children and controls recognize an identical collection of linear epitopes of alpha-gliadin. Clin Exp Immunol 114: 189–195

Tuohy VK, Yu M, Ling Y, Kawczak JA, Kinkel RP (1999) Spontaneous regression of primary auto-reactivity during chronic progression of experimental autoimmune encephalitis and multiple sclerosis. J Exp Med 189: 1033–1042

van de Wal Y, Kooy YM, van Veelen P, Vader W, August SA, Drijfhout JW, Pena SA, Koning F (1999) Glutenin is involved in the gluten-driven mucosal T cell response. Eur J Immunol 29: 3133–3139

Weiser H (1995) The precipitating factor in coeliac disease. Ballieres Clin Gastroenterol 9: 191–207

Yewdell JW, Bennink JR (1999) Immunodominance in major histocompatibility complex class I-restricted T lymphocyte responses. Annu Rev Immunol 17: 51–88

On the extrapolation from animal models to human disease for the design of immunotherapy in autoimmune diabetes

Jean-François Bach*

Maladies Auto-immunes, Unité de Institut National de la Santé et de la Recherche Médicale,
Hôpital Necker, Paris, France

Introduction

Type 1 diabetes, insulin-dependent diabetes mellitus (IDDM) is a T-cell-mediated autoimmune disease (Bach 1994). It is thus logical to attempt to stop or better prevent disease progression by immunotherapy. A multitude of immunological treatments have been shown to be successful in the most currently available model of type 1 diabetes, namely, the nonobese diabetic (NOD) mouse. This observation may be taken in a positive fashion, paving the way for testing these strategies in humans. Conversely, one may wonder whether the NOD mouse is not, in some ways, "too sensitive" to immunological intervention, rendering the extrapolation of results obtained in NOD mice to human diabetes uncertain. This is, in fact, a very complex question which shall be addressed in some detail below.

Immunotherapy in NOD mice

A wide array of methods has been shown to prevent diabetes onset in NOD mice. Table 1 provides a probably nonexhaustive list of compounds or methods reported to have been effective. Today, one may enumerate more than 160 methods. Some of these methods, such as bone marrow allogeneic transplantation following irradiation or depleting anti-T-cell monoclonal antibodies, are somewhat aggressive. Others are relatively mild, such as oral administration of nonpathogenic lactobacilli or vitamin D3. Points arguing in favor or against the potential significance of these methods in the context of their application to the immunotherapy of human IDDM will be presented.

* Author's address: INSERM U25, Hôpital Necker, 161 rue de Sèvres, 75743 Paris Cedex 15, France.
E-mail: bach@necker.fr

Table 1. Compounds or methods reported to be effective in preventing diabetes in the NOD mouse

T cell depletion or sequestration/diversion
Depletion
  Anti-CD3
  Anti-CD4
  Anti-CD8
  Anti-CD44
  Anti-CD45RA
  Anti-CD45RB
  Anti-Thy 1.2
  Anti-lymphocyte globulin
  Neonatal thymectomy
Sequestration/diversion
  Anti-CD43
  Anti-VLA-1
  Anti-VLA-4
  VLA-4-Ig fusion protein
  Anti-CD62L

Blockade of T cell activation
Chemical immunosuppressants
  Cyclosporin A
  FK506
  Azathioprine
  Rapamycin
  Deoxyspergualin
Gamma irradiation

TCR targeting
TCR$\alpha\beta$ antibody
CD3 antibody
Vβ8 antibody
T cell vaccination
  Polyclonal activated T cells
  Glutaraldehyde-treated T cells
  Activated T cells
  Vβ8 T cells
  Anti hsp60 T cell clone
Blocking peptides

Targeting of MHC molecule
Anti-class I
Anti-class II
MHC transgenic mice (class I, I-A, I-E)

Costimulation and adhesion
Costimulation molecules
  Anti-CD28
  CTLA4-Ig
  Anti-B7.2
  Anti-CD40 L
Adhesion molecules
  Anti-ICAM-1

Soluble ICAM-1
Recombinant protein
Gene therapy
Anti-Mac
Anti-LFA-1

Cytokine blockade
IFN-γ
  Anti-IFN-γ
  IFNγR-Ig
IL-2
  Anti-IL-2 R
  IL-2 R-Ig fusion protein
  IL-2 diphtheria toxin protein
IL-12
  Anti-IL-12
  IL-12 antagonist (p40)2
INFα (oral)
IL-1
  IL-1 antibody
  IL-1 antagonist
IL-6
Lymphotoxin receptor

Pharmacologically active cytokines
IL-4
IL-10
IL-13
IL-3
G-CSF
Lymphotoxin
IL-11
IL-1α
TNF-α

Tolerance to soluble β cell autoantigens
Insulin
  Oral
  Oral + IL-10
  Intranasal
  Subcutaneous
    Native protein
    B chain
  Inactive analog
  DNA vaccination
  Gene transfer delivery
  (proinsulin gene)
  Cholera toxin conjugate
Glutamic acid decarboxylase (GAD)
  Oral
  Intranasal
  Subcutaneous

Intrathymic
DNA vaccination
Anti-GAD antibody
Heat shock protein 60 (hsp 60)
  Subcutaneous–intraperitoneal
  Protein
  P277 peptide
  Gene transfer delivery
Pancreatic extracts (oral)

Stimulation of regulatory T cells
Pathogens
  Bacteria
    Mycobacteria (*M. bovis*, *M. avium*, CFA)
    Lactobacillus casei
    Streptococcal extract
    Klebsiella extract
    E. coli (+ oral insulin)
  Viruses
    mouse hepatitis virus
    lactate dehydrogenase-elevating virus
    lymphocytic choriomeningitis virus
  Parasites
    Filariae
    Schistosoma
Stimulation of innate immunity
(α galactosylceramide)
Nondepleting anti-T cell antibodies
  Anti-CD3
  Anti-CD4
  Superantigens

Gene therapy
β Cell antigens
  DNA vaccination
  GAD Ig
IL-4
  Retrovirus (T cell transfection)
  Biolistic
  Adenovirus
  IL-4 IgG1
IL-10
  T cell transfection
  Local
  Systemic
ICAM-1
IFN-γR-IgGl
TGF-β
Calcitonin

Cell therapy
Islet or segmental pancreas transplantation
(+ immunosuppression)

Syngeneic
Allogeneic
Intrathymic islet transplantation
Bone marrow transplantation
  Allogeneic
  Syngeneic
Dendritic cells
NK T cells
CD4 cell lines
  Polyclonal
  Anti-Ia^{g7}
Allogeneic cells
  Macrophages
  Spleen cells

Inhibition of β cell lesion
Nicotinamide
Antioxidants
  Vitamin E
  Probucol analog
  Probucol + deflazacort
  Aminoguanidine
Anti-inflammatory agents
  Pentoxiphyllin
  Rolipram

Miscellaneous
Immunomodulators
  Linomide
  Ling-zhi-8
  D-glucan
  Multifunctional protein 14
  Ciamexon
  Cholerotoxin B
  Vanadate
  Vitamin D3 analogue
Hormones and related proteins
  Androgens
  IGF-1
Immunomanipulation
  Natural antibodies
  Lupus idiotype
  LPS
Diet (casein hydrolysate)
Other
  Sulfatide
  Bee venom
  Kampo formulation
  Silica
  Ganglioside
  Anti-asialo GM-1 antibody
  Hyaluronidase
  Concanavalin A

Arguments against extrapolation from the model

Differences between NOD mouse and human diabetes

Diabetes is more common in female than in male NOD mice, a gender difference not found in human IDDM except in the type 1b form (associated with extra-pancreatic autoantibodies). A large variety of non-β-cell-specific autoimmune manifestations are found in NOD mice and not in the majority of IDDM patients, except again the 10% of type 1b patients. The autoantibody profile shows important differences with a much higher prevalence of anti-GAD and anti-IA-2 in humans than in mice (Bach 1998). In fact, the major difference between NOD mice and human type 1 diabetes, which most probably explains the differences just mentioned, is that the disease is heterogeneous in humans, whereas NOD mice are all multiple copies of a single individual, and additionally homozygous at all loci, like any inbred mouse strain. The difference also applies at the level of environmental factors, which are extremely heterogeneous in humans, but very similar for all mice in a given colony.

Differences in the timing of treatment staging of IDDM

NOD mice are genetically predisposed to becoming diabetic. One can thus start treatment at any age before the initiation of the pathogenic autoimmune process. This is hardly feasible in humans. In most cases, patients will show up and be treated when the disease is declared. Thanks to prediction markers (essentially β-cell-specific antibodies), one may treat prediabetics, but even these individuals are already relatively advanced in the disease process, since they produce sufficient amounts of β-cell-specific autoantibodies to be detectable in the blood (Bach 1994). Trials should be performed in mice and humans under comparable timing conditions. This is a critical point since only a very few of the more than 160 methods listed in Table 1 are still active in mice older than 16–18 weeks and even fewer when clinical diabetes has begun (Table 2).

It may be worth mentioning that the following three variants of the NOD model used for a number of drugs, which are often considered as tests for late intervention, are not so clearly understood.

Table 2. Methods active at a late age in NOD mice

Agent	Activity of agent at time of:		Reference
	>16 weeks of age	Declared diabetes	
Heat shock protein 60	+		Elias and Cohen 1994
Anti-CD4 + anti CD8		+	Maki et al. 1992
Anti-CD3		+	Chatenoud et al. 1994
Antilymphocyte serum		+	Maki et al. 1992
Soluble ICAM-1 (gene therapy)		+	Bertry-Coussot et al. 2002

Table 3. Examples of agents active on three late-intervention variants of the NOD mouse model

Model variant	Agent
Cyclophosphamide-induced diabetes	CD3 antibody, BCG, α-GalCer
Diabetes transfer in irradiated or scid mice	CD4 antibody, IFNγ antibody
Diabetes relapse in islet grafted mice	CD4 antibody, CD3 antibody, α-GalCer, GAD

Cyclophosphamide-induced diabetes is a fulminant form of the disease (Yasunami and Bach 1988). However, it appears that although the disease evolves rapidly, it probably progresses through all stages of the disease, with an initial cytotoxic β-cell lesion (induced by the alkylating agent) and a selective destruction of regulatory T cells.

In diabetes transfer to irradiated or scid NOD mice, spleen cells from overtly diabetic mice are used which are fully differentiated β-cell-specific T cells (Miller et al. 1988). It remains, though, that it takes several weeks before the pool of effector cells builds up to a size sufficient to induce destructive insulitis following a series of events which might also involve the entire process of diabetogenesis.

In the prevention of diabetes recurrence in diabetic NOD mice grafted with syngeneic islets (Wang et al. 1987) the problem is the absence of normal vasculature (the islet grafts are placed under the kidney capsule).

In fact, it is interesting to note that many agents acting in these three models (Table 3) lose their activity at late stages in the spontaneous animal model.

Efficacy of mild treatments

It may appear surprising to see that a severe and devastating disease such as IDDM may be prevented in NOD mice by treatments as simple as bee venom (Kim et al. 1999), pentoxyfilline (Liang et al. 1998), or streptococcal extracts (Toyota et al. 1986). The observation of such effects has cast doubts on the validity of the NOD model. Looking closely at the data, it appears that the prevention is usually partial and transient, and that the effect is only obtained when the treatment is applied at a very young age. It would be interesting to know whether the same effects might be obtained in humans, for example, very young children at risk of developing diabetes a very long time before their putative start of the disease. One can certainly not exclude the possibility that these mild treatments might work. It would, after all, be in keeping with the chaos theory that the progression to severe autoimmunity is a very long process, beginning in a very progressive fashion, with a long period of benign autoimmunity, most sensitive to intervention.

Therapeutic effect of a short-duration treatment

Several of the methods discussed above are fully efficient even when they are only administered over a very short period of time, a single injection of hsp60 (Elias and Cohen 1994) or 5 days for CD3 antibody (Chatenoud et al. 1994). This may be surprising in view of the chronicity of the autoimmune process just discussed. Two orders of factors may explain the phenomenon. Firstly, some of the methods used induce an active biological process and, as for vaccination, a single-shot trigger suffices. Secondly, restoration of immunoregulation, which is a central mechanism for many of the methods in question, can have a "snowball effect". In other words, regulation promotes regulation in an autocrine fashion. This has been well demonstrated for Th2 cells where cytokines produced by these cells are autocrine growth factors, notably interleukin-4.

Arguments supporting the model

Close similarity to human disease

In spite of minor differences, the NOD mouse disease closely resembles human disease (Bach 1994). Insulitis progression is similar at all stages. Predisposition genes appear similar as far as one can tell, notably for MHC genes. The role of environment is also apparently similar for exacerbating factors (e.g., coxsackie viruses) and for protective ones (particularly infections) (Bach 2001). The NOD homogeneity, which remains the major difference from the human disease, as discussed above, is, in fact, a crucial experimental advantage insofar as it provides a major statistical power which is lacking in humans.

Good predictive value for drug testing

A number of products have been submitted to clinical trials in human type 1 diabetes, either in recently diagnosed diabetes or in prediabetes (Table 4). All have

Table 4. Drugs tested in human diabetes

Stage of diabetes and administered agent	Effect of agent	Reference(s)
Prediabetes		
Parenteral insulin	negative	Diabetes Prevention Trial-Type 1 Diabetes Study Group 2002
Nicotinamide	negative	Lampeter et al. 1998
Recently diagnosed diabetes		
Cyclosporin A	positive	Canadian-European Randomized Control Trial Group 1988, Feutren et al. 1986
Azathioprine + steroids	positive	Silverstein et al. 1988
Nicotinamide	partially positive	Pozzilli et al. 1989
hsp 60	positive	Raz et al. 2001
CD3 antibody	positive	Herold et al. 2002

been shown to prevent diabetes onset in the NOD mouse. Only CD3 antibody (Chatenoud et al. 1994) and hsp60 (Elias and Cohen 1994) have been shown to act at a late stage. It is reassuring to see that precisely these two products have recently been shown to slow down diabetes progression in recently diagnosed patients after administration of a short-duration treatment along the lines of the protocols used in NOD mice (Raz et al. 2001, Herold et al. 2002).

Accessibility to mechanisms

One of the major advantages of the NOD mouse model is the access to mechanisms of the therapeutic effect. It is remarkable to see how much information has been gained in NOD mice on the mode of action of drugs such as parenteral or oral insulin or GAD, CD3 antibody, or BCG (Bach and Chatenoud 2001). This is of invaluable help in guiding protocol selection and thinking of drug combinations.

Conclusions

Drug testing in animal models represents a necessary phase in drug development. The validity of the model for extrapolation to humans is often questioned, notably in cancer treatment. The NOD mouse has been used for an unusually large number of methods. The high success rate has led to questioning the model. The arguments discussed above provide a fair response to some of these questions. When used under the strict conditions of the clinical presentation of diabetic patients, notably in terms of disease stage, the NOD mouse appears to be a very good predictive model. Results must, however, be interpreted with caution. Placebo-controlled, well-designed, randomized trials which can validate a product are expensive in terms of time, energy, and money. They should only be initiated after careful analysis of data obtained in NOD mice, in terms of the remarks developed above.

References

Bach J-F (1994) Insulin-dependent diabetes mellitus as an autoimmune disease. Endocrine Rev 15: 516–542

Bach J-F (1998) The natural history of islet-specific autoimmunity in NOD mice. In: Leiter E, Atkinson M (eds) NOD mice and related strains: research applications in diabetes, AIDS, cancer and other diseases. RG Landes, Austin, Tex, pp 121–144

Bach J-F (2001) Protective role of infections and vaccinations on autoimmune diseases. J Autoimmun 16: 347–353

Bach J-F, Chatenoud L (2001) Tolerance to islet autoantigens and type I diabetes. Annu Rev Immunol 19: 131–161

Bertry-Coussot L, Lucas B, Danel Claire, Halbwachs-Mecarelli L, Bach J-F, Chatenoud L, Lemarchand P (2002) Long-term reversal of established autoimmunity upon transient blockade of the LFA-1/inter-cellular adhesion molecule-1 pathway. J Immunol 168: 3641–3648

Canadian-European Randomized Control Trial Group (1988) Cyclosporin-induced remission of IDDM after early intervention: association of 1 yr of cyclosporin treatment with enhanced insulin secretion. Diabetes 37: 1574–1582

Chatenoud L, Thervet E, Primo J, Bach J-F (1994) Anti-CD3 antibody induces long-term remission of overt autoimmunity in nonobese diabetic mice. Proc Natl Acad Sci USA 91: 123–127

Diabetes Prevention Trial-Type 1 Diabetes Study Group (2002) Effects of insulin in relatives of patients with type 1 diabetes mellitu. N Engl J Med 346: 1685–1691

Elias D, Cohen IR (1994) Peptide therapy for diabetes in NOD mice. Lancet 343: 704–706

Feutren G, Papoz L, Assan R, Vialettes B, Karsenty G, Vexiau P, Du Rostu H, Rodier M, Sirmai J, Lallemand A, Bach J-F (1986) Cyclosporin increases the rate and length of remissions in insulin-dependent diabetes of recent onset: results of a multicentre double-blind trial. Lancet 2: 119–124

Herold KC, Hagopian W, Auger JA, Poumian-Ruiz E, Taylor L, Donaldson D, Gitelman SE, Harlan DM, Xu D, Zivin RA, Bluestone JA (2002) Anti-CD3 monoclonal antibody in new-onset type 1 diabetes mellitus. N Engl J Med 346: 1692–1698

Kim JY, Cho SH, Kim YW, Jang EC, Park SY, Kim EJ, Lee SK (1999) Effects of BCG, lymphotoxin and bee venom on insulitis and development of IDDM in non-obese diabetic mice. J Kor Med Sci 14: 648–652

Lampeter EF, Klinghammer A, Scherbaum WA, Heinze E, Haastert B, Giani G, Kolb H (1998) The Deutsche Nicotinamide Intervention Study: an attempt to prevent type 1 diabetes: DENIS Group. Diabetes 47: 980–984

Liang L, Beshay E, Prud'Homme GJ (1998) The phosphodiesterase inhibitors pentoxifylline and rolipram prevent diabetes in NOD mice. Diabetes 47: 570–575

Maki T, Ichikawa T, Blanco R, Porter J (1992) Long-term abrogation of autoimmune diabetes in nonobese diabetic mice by immunotherapy with anti-lymphocyte serum. Proc Natl Acad Sci USA 89: 3434–3438

Miller BJ, Appel MC, O'Neil JJ, Wicker LS (1988) Both the Lyt-2$^+$ and L3T4$^+$ T cell subsets are required for the transfer of diabetes in nonobese diabetic mice. J Immunol 140: 52–58

Pozzilli P, Visalli N, Ghirlanda G, Manna R, Andreani D (1989) Nicotinamide increases C-peptide secretion in patients with recent onset type 1 diabetes. Diabet Med 6: 568–572

Raz I, Elias D, Avron A, Tamir M, Metzger M, Cohen IR (2001) Beta-cell function in new-onset type 1 diabetes and immunomodulation with a heat-shock protein peptide (DiaPep277): a randomised, double-blind, phase II trial. Lancet 358: 1749–1753

Silverstein J, MacLaren N, Riley W, Spillar R, Radjenovic D, Johnson S (1988) Immunosuppression with azathioprine and prednisone in recent-onset insulin-dependent diabetes mellitus. N Engl J Med 319: 599–604

Toyota T, Satoh J, Oya K, Shintani S, Okano T (1986) Streptococcal preparation (OK-432) inhibits development of type I diabetes in NOD mice. Diabetes 35: 496–499

Wang Y, Hao L, Gill RG, Lafferty KJ (1987) Autoimmune diabetes in NOD mouse is L3T4 T-lymphocyte dependent. Diabetes 36: 535–538

Yasunami R, Bach J-F (1988) Anti-suppressor effect of cyclophosphamide on the development of spontaneous diabetes in NOD mice. Eur J Immunol 18: 481–484

Use of olfactory ensheathing cells as candidates for transplant-mediated repair of central nervous system lesions

Susan C. Barnett*

Departments of Neurology and Medical Oncology, University of Glasgow,
Glasgow, United Kingdom

Introduction

The rat olfactory system is a tissue of extreme interest. It has the capacity to support axonal outgrowth throughout the life of the animal and more specifically can maintain continual growth of olfactory axons during natural turnover and also after injury. These newly generated neurons originate from stem cells present in the olfactory epithelium and extend axons which can penetrate into the adult central nervous system (CNS) tissue and resynapse with the second-order axons present at the glomerolus in the olfactory bulb (Doucette 1984, Farbman 1990, Raisman 1985). It is thought that this property is in part due to the specialized glial cells that ensheath the olfactory neurons and reside in the olfactory bulb and nerve known as olfactory ensheathing cells (OECs) (Fig. 1).

Recently, OECs have attracted much interest as candidate cell for transplantation-mediated repair of CNS lesions (see reviews by Franklin and Barnett 2000, Raisman 2001) due to their ability to remyelinate axons in demyelinating lesions (Franklin et al. 1996, Imaizumi et al. 1998) and support regrowth of transected axons (Ramon-Cueto and Nieto-Sampedro 1994, Smale et al. 1996) as well as seemingly support functional recovery of these axons after transplantation (Imaizumi et al. 2000, Li et al. 1997, Navarro et al. 1999, Ramon-Cueto et al. 2000). The excitement surrounding the concept that OECs are candidates for use in the clinic for therapy in the repair of CNS lesions is fuelled by the remarkable functional recovery described in rats which have received a transplantation of rOECs after

* Author's address: Department of Neurology, University of Glasgow, Switchback Road, Glasgow G61 1BD, United Kingdom.
E-mail: gpma37@udcf.gla.ac.uk

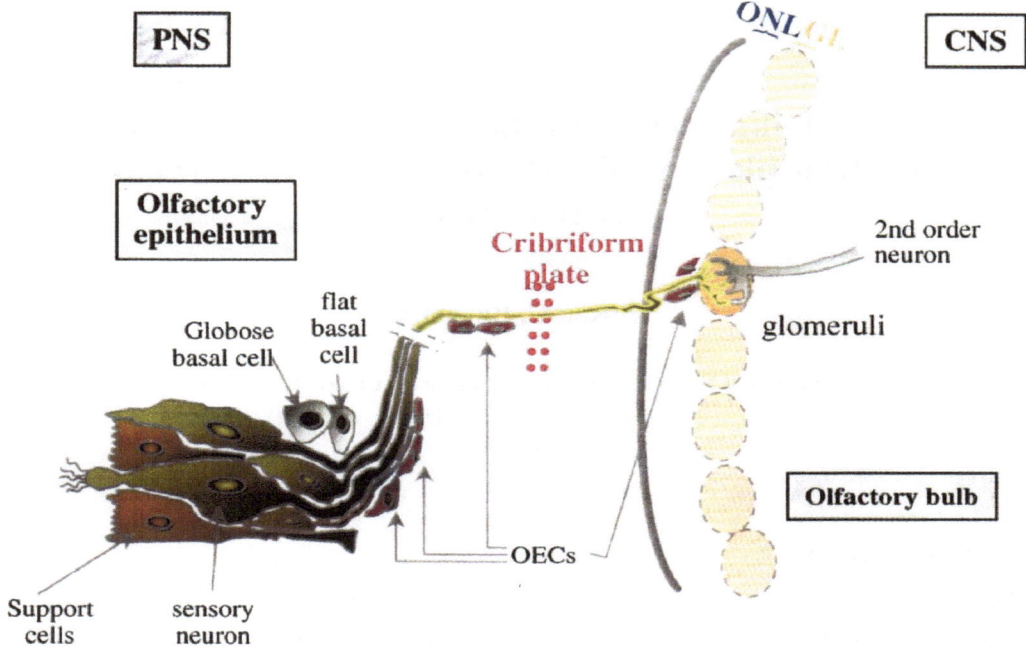

Fig. 1. Scheme of the rat olfactory system. The olfactory nerves are generated from stem cells in the epithelium, which course through the cribriform plate and enter the olfactory nerve layer (*ONL*) of the olfactory bulb. In the second layer of the bulb, the glomerular layer (*GL*), the olfactory nerves synapse with the second-order neurons in the glomeruli. Bundles of unmyelinated nerves are ensheathed by the glial cells (*OECs*). The interest for this tissue is the ability of the glial cells to coexist in both peripheral nervous system (epithelium) and central nervous system tissues (bulb) and to support axonal outgrowth throughout the life

either a complete transection of their spinal cord (Ramon-Cueto et al. 2000, Navarro et al. 1999) or after transection of the corticospinal tract (Li et al. 1997).

Cell biological characteristics of rat OECs

Our previous studies on the rat olfactory bulb have identified two classes of OECs defined as Schwann cell-like and astrocytelike (Franceschini and Barnett 1996) and similar cell types have been identified in the olfactory nerve (Pixley 1992). The cells are purified from the olfactory bulb of perinatal rat pups with the fluorescence-activated cell sorter (FACS) and the O4 antibody and anti-galacto-cerboside (Barnett et al. 1993a, b) (Fig. 2). In our studies, O4-positive FACS-purified OECs placed in serum-free culture medium (DMEM-BS; Bottenstein et al. 1979) conditioned by astrocytes (ACM, astrocyte-conditioned medium; Noble and Murray 1984) develop into the two OEC subtypes (Franceschini and Barnett 1996). ACM is a well-known source of many mitogens used in the growth of other glial cells (Noble and Murray 1984). These OEC subtypes are classified by their expression of the Schwann cell markers, low-affinity nerve growth factor

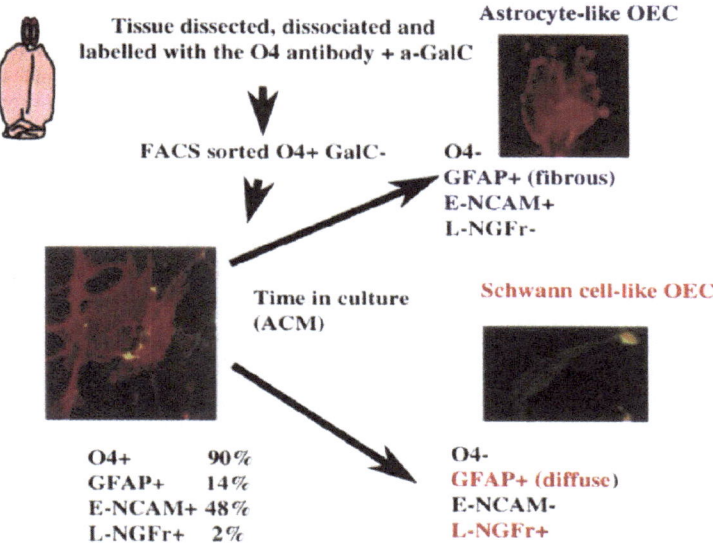

Fig. 2. Scheme for the purification of the two rOECs subtypes. 7-day-old rat olfactory bulbs were dissected and enzymatically dissociated with collagenase. The cell suspension was incubated with the O4 antibody and anti-galctocerebroside (GalC) for 1 h on ice and then washed twice, resuspended in the fluorescein- and phycoerythrin-conjugated secondary antibodies and incubated on ice for a further 45 min. After two washes the cells were sorted with a FACS as an O4-positive and GalC-negative cell population. This selects against committed oligodendrocytes that express the myelin marker GalC. Cells were placed in culture incubated in ACM and refed three times a week. After around 3 weeks in culture the Schwann cell-like and astrocytelike OEC can be identified by their differing expression of L-NGFr and E-NCAM and the variability in GFAP intensity. Detailed methods can be found in Barnett et al. (1993a, b)

receptor (L-NGFr, P75) and diffuse glial fibrillary acidic protein (GFAP) expression, or the astrocyte markers, fibrous GFAP and the embryonic form of neural cell adhesion molecule (E-NCAM), which is the polysialylated isoform of NCAM. E-NCAM has been identified on cells that in adult life retain embryonic-like features, for example, the astrocytes in the hypothalamo-neurohypophysial systems (Bonfanti et al. 1992). E-NCAM has been associated with decreasing the adhesive properties of N-CAM, thus permitting the cellular rearrangements characterizing neurohistogenesis and plasticity (Bonfanti et al. 1993, Muller and O'Rahilly 1990, Seki and Rutishauser 1998, Theodosis et al. 1999). In CNS repair the two antigenic subtypes may have different roles (Raisman 2001) with the expression of L-NGFr on their surface as a means of presenting the tropic and trophic support to the regenerating olfactory axons (Ramon-Cueto et al. 1993) and E-NCAM expression used for directing the axons to their correct position.

Growth factor requirements of rat OECs

Initial studies on the growth conditions for rOECs used Dulbecco modified Eagle medium containing 10% foetal calf serum (DMEM-FCS) as the OEC mitogen (Ramon-Cueto et al. 1993, Li et al. 1998). This could support the growth of OECs for several weeks, although growth was limited (Raisman 2001, Yan et al. 2001) and did not support the identification of the two OEC subtypes (Barnett and Franceschini 1999). Initially, we found that conditioned medium from cortical type-1 astrocytes was a potent mitogen and survival factor for OECs (Barnett et al. 1993), which later we discovered to be a beta isoform of the neuregulin family of proteins (Pollock et al. 1999). Recently it has been shown that the combination of forskolin, neuregulin, and FGF2 is a potent OEC mitogen for adult OECs (Yin et al. 2000). However, these studies did not examine the proliferation rate of the OECs past 6 days nor did they examine the differentiation status of OECs in these four mitogens. Recently, we have shown that OECs can proliferate at a faster rate and for a longer time (past 9 weeks) if they are incubated in those four mitogens diluted in ACM (Alexander et al. 2002). Interestingly in this study we show that ACM induces a proliferation arrest in the OECs that is reversible by a mix of forskolin, neuregulin, and FGF2 (known as olfactory mitogen medium, OMM) diluted in ACM (OMM/ACM). Once these cells were arrested for 2 weeks in ACM and then incubated in ACM/OMM, the resulting growth factor response rate to OMM/ACM was longer and the modulation of the two OEC-specific markers, L-NGFr and E-NCAM, was different compared to cells treated in these factors without the growth arrest. Treatment of OECs with OMM diluted in minimal DMEM medium (DMEM-BS; Bottenstein and Sato 1979) termed DMEM-BS/OMM, supported the expression of L-NGFr, O4, and E-NCAM compared to L-NGFr, O4, and very little E-NCAM when grown in OMM/ACM. These studies illustrate the plastic nature of the OECs with the variability in their expression of the three markers O4, L-NGFr, and E-NCAM.

The plasticity of the OEC subtypes in vitro has also been shown in vivo (Franklin et al. 1996). In these studies a clonal OEC cell line was transplanted into a persistently demyelinated CNS lesion of the rat spinal cord. This is a well-documented model system for demyelination in the CNS (Blakemore et al. 1990, 1994, 1995; Blakemore and Franklin 1991; Franklin and Blakemore 1998). Repair to the denuded axons could only come from the injected transplant cells, and in these experiments we found that the axons were myelinated with peripheral nervous system type myelin, therefore demonstrating the presence of the Schwann cell-like OEC. In addition, a second cell type could be detected in the lesion that did not ensheath the axon but had the phenotype of an astrocytelike OEC, expressing abundant GFAP filaments throughout the cytoplasm (Franklin et al. 1996).

Do antigenically equivalent OEC exist in human tissue?

For the use of OECs as a therapeutic approach for the repair of human CNS damage to become a reality, it will be necessary to obtain human olfactory ensheathing cells (hOECs). A key issue remains whether cells similar to those obtained from the rat exist in the olfactory tissue of humans, a mammal that has a relatively poorly developed sense of smell. It has been suggested from an immunohistochemical study using the antibody to olfactory marker protein (OMP) that there is continuous cell turnover in the neurons of the human olfactory neuroepithelium (Nakashima et al. 1985) and from scanning electron microscopy (Moran et al.

1982, Morrison and Costanzo 1990, Nakashima et al. 1984) and tissue culture studies (Lu et al. 2001) that support cells analogous to glia within the CNS are present in the human olfactory epithelium. However, it is not clear whether the two classes of OECs which have been described for the rat are present in the olfactory epithelium and bulb since a direct comparison using the markers that define the rat cells has not been carried out (Barber and Dahl 1987, Barnett et al. 1993, Franceschini and Barnett 1996, Pixley 1992, Ramon-Cueto et al. 1993).

From tissue collected by the U.K. MS Tissue Bank at Charing Cross Hospital (post-mortem delay of 7.5–17 h), we have identified cells with immunological properties similar to rat OECs (Barnett et al. 2000) (Fig. 3). Cell suspensions have been made from olfactory bulb or nerve tissue taken during surgery when removal was a necessary part of normal surgical procedures and these cells label with the L-NGFr and express properties very similar to the Schwann cell-like OECs (Barnett et al. 2000). However, it is clear that if these cells are not purified before use there will be an outgrowth of contaminating cells. In this study we found that although during the first 7 days in cultures the L-NGFr-positive hOECs grew well in medium containing 10% FCS, so did contaminating endothelial cells, fibroblasts, and other nonglial cell types (Barnett et al. 2000). Initial identification of the optimal growth factor conditions for the growth of hOECs suggests that they respond in a manner similar to rOECs and grow in conditioned medium from astrocytes or 10 ng of heregulin β1 per ml (Franceschini and Barnett 1996, Pollock et al. 1999, Barnett et al. 2000). Purified cultures of hOECs can be obtained by

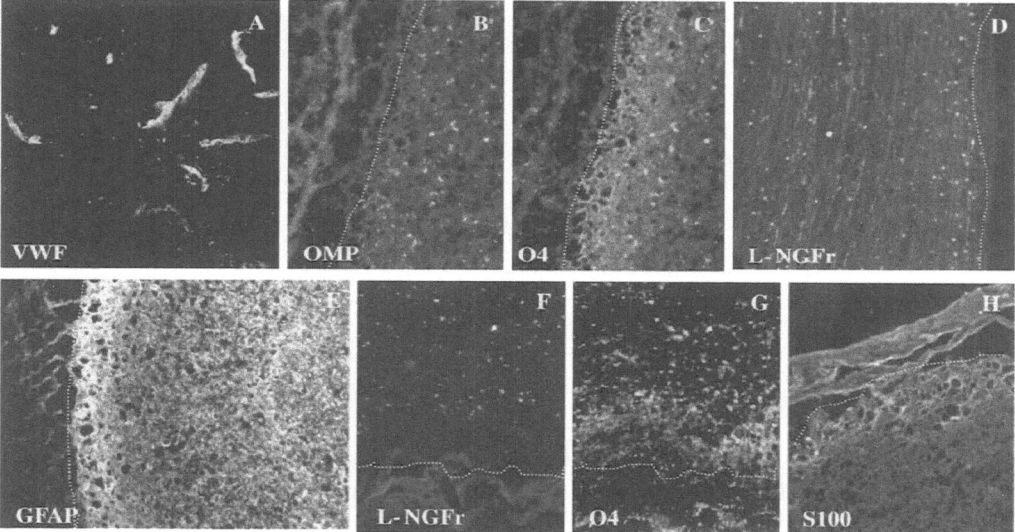

Fig. 3A–H. Immunohistochemistry of human olfactory bulbs. Longitudinal sections of the olfactory bulb illustrating the outer olfactory nerve layer and the glomerular layer of the olfactory bulb. **A** Von Willebrand factor-positive endothelial cells of blood vessels are present in the center of the bulb. **B** Immunoreactivity with anti-OMP. **C–H** The outer layer of the olfactory bulb expressed immunoreactivity with the O4 antibody (**C** and **G**), anti-L-NGFr (**D** and **F**), anti-GFAP (**E**), and anti-S100 (**H**), markers typical of rat OECs. Dotted lines represent the edge of the bulb. ×242

immunopanning using the L-NGFr antibody, FACS sorting, or using magnetic beads coupled to antibodies. In the latter situation we have obtained enriched cultures of hOECs (Barnett et al. 2000). Using our purified hOECs, which are between 50–70% L-NGFr positive, we have shown that they can effect transplant-mediated remyelination of demyelinated rat CNS axons (Barnett et al. 2000). In these experiments a lesion was created in the spinal cord of adult rats by injecting a gliotoxin and this region of spinal cord was irradiated so as to prevent the host glia from repopulating the denuded axons (Blakemore et al. 1990, 1994, 1995; Blakemore and Franklin 1991; Franklin and Blakemore 1998). Confirmation of our results with nonpurified hOECs has also been demonstrated (Kato et al. 2000). This is exciting data as it shows that the hOEC not only exhibits cellular properties of the rOEC but also can carry out more physiological roles.

With the recent identification of ACM/OMM as a potent rOEC mitogen we have looked into the ability of hOECs to respond to these conditions (Fig. 4). In fact, these conditions are mitogenic, but not as mitogenic as ACM. Cells can be identified in these factors by the characteristics of rOECs, namely, expressing O4, E-NCAM, and L-NGFr (Fig. 5). It appears that ACM/OMM is not as potent a mitogen as ACM and that there clearly are differences in the growth factor responses between rat and human OECs.

Studies of the cellular and molecular properties of OECs are still in their infancy. It is clear that there are at least two OECs subtypes, and that nonpurified preparations can still effect functional recovery. This leaves open the idea that it

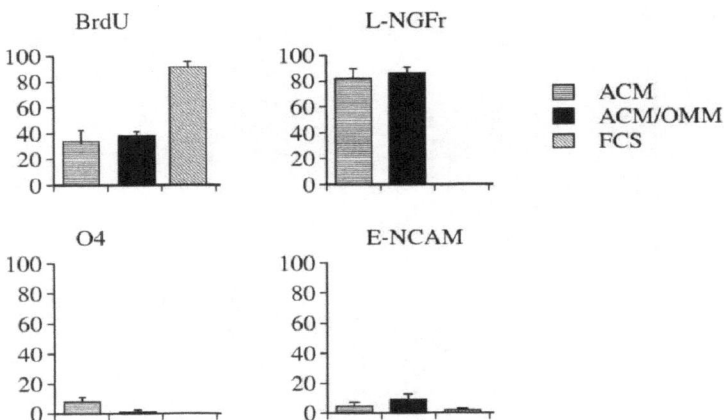

Fig. 4. Summary of bromodeoxyuridine (BrdU) uptake and antigenic phenotype of human OECs. Cells were placed on coverslips immediately after enzymatic dissociation from a human olfactory bulb. They were incubated in ACM (1:5 dilution), ACM/OMM, or DMEM-FCS for 2 weeks and then immunolabelled with BrdU after preincubation overnight with 20 µM BrdU to measure cells in the S phase of the cell cycle and therefore proliferation. Using 4′,6-diamidino-2-phenylindole to mark the nuclei, the O4 antibody, anti-E-NCAM, and anti-L-NGFr, and indirect immunofluorescence, we assessed the antigenic phenotype of the resulting cells. Although cell proliferation was greatest in DMEM-FCS, the majority of the cells did not label with the OEC markers and represent the outgrowth of contaminating cells. In the other serum-free culture conditions, most of the cells labelled with L-NGFr, but only a few expressed O4 or E-NCAM. Methods can be found in Barnett et al. (2000) and Alexander et al. (2002)

ACM   ACM/OMM   FCS

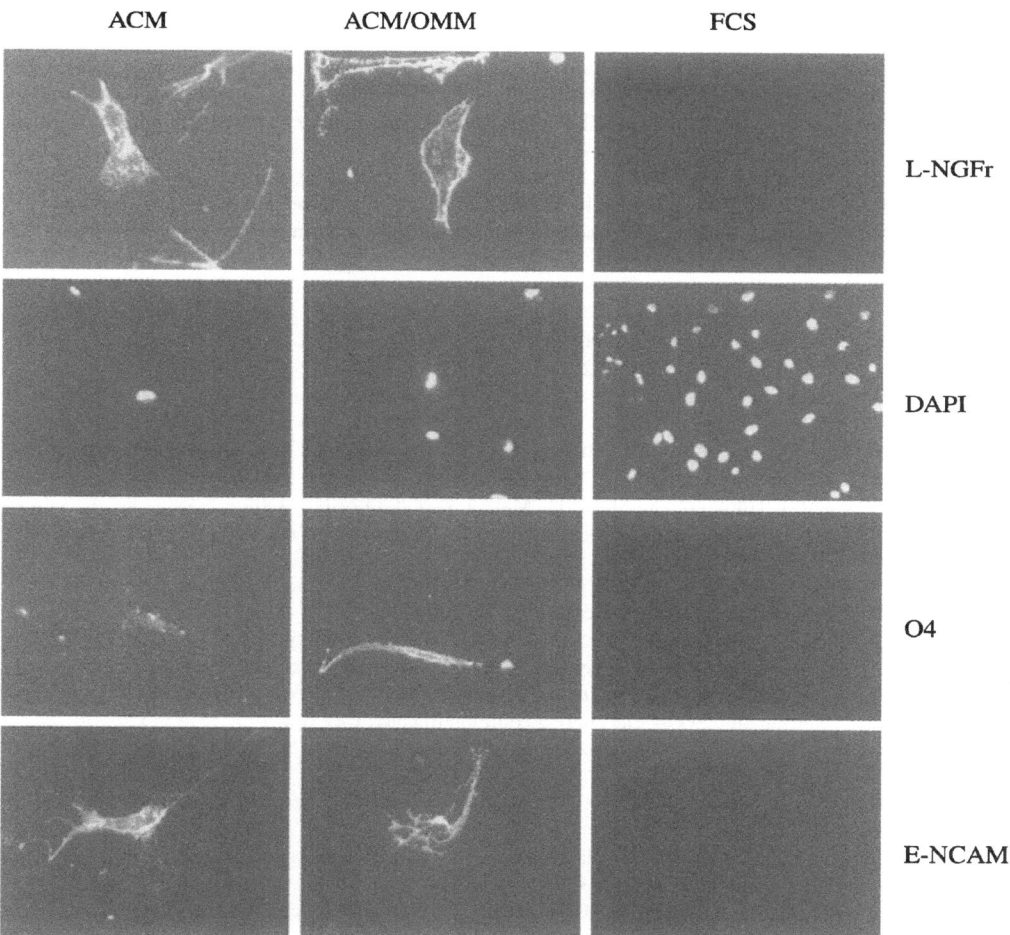

L-NGFr

DAPI

O4

E-NCAM

Fig. 5. Immunocytochemistry of human OECs. The cells were cultured and grown in ACM, ACM/OMM, or DMEM-FCS as described in the legend of Fig. 4 and were immunolabelled with the O4 antibody, anti-L-NGFr, and anti-E-NCAM. It can be seen that very few OECs exist in DMEM-FCS. L-NGFr is the major marker with occasional cells expressing the O4 antibody and E-NCAM. ×400

is not a single cell type that repairs the lesions but a mixture of cell types. Future work should be able to clarify the functional role of the different cell types that make up the olfactory system in the repair of CNS lesions and bring us closer to the use of the hOEC in the repair of CNS lesions.

References

Alexander CL, FitzGerald UF, Barnett SC (2002) Identification of growth factors that promote long-term proliferation of olfactory ensheathing cells and modulate their antigenic phenotype. Glia 37: 349–364
Barber PC, Dahl D (1987) Glial fibrillary acidic protein (GFAP)-like immunoreactivity in normal and transected rat olfactory nerve. Exp Brain Res 65: 681–685

Barnett SC (1993) The culture of central nervous system (CNS) glial cells. In: Freshney IR (ed) Culture of animal cells, 3rd edn. Wiley-Liss, New York, pp 337–341

Barnett SC, Franceschini IA (1999) Adhesion molecule expression and phenotype of glial cells in the olfactory tract. Adv Exp Med Biol 468: 297–307

Barnett SC, Hutchins AM, Noble M (1993) Purification of olfactory nerve ensheathing cells from the olfactory bulb. Dev Biol 155: 337–350

Barnett SC, Alexander CL, Gilson J, Clark L, Dunn L, Papanastassiou V, Kennedy PGE, Ishwashita Y, Franklin RJM (2000) Identification of the human olfactory ensheathing cell (OEC) and demonstration of its ability to remyelinate experimentally-induced demyelinating lesions in the rat spinal cord. Brain 123: 101–108

Blakemore WF, Franklin RJM (1991) Transplantation of glial cells into the CNS. Trends Neurosci 14: 323–327

Blakemore WF, Crang AJ, Franklin RJ (1990) Transplantation of glial cell cultures into areas of demyelination in the adult CNS. Prog Brain Res 82: 225–232

Blakemore WF, Franklin RJ, Crang AJ (1994) Repair of demyelinated lesions by glial cell transplantation. J Neurol 242: S61–S63

Blakemore WF, Olby NJ, Franklin RJM (1995) The use of transplanted glial cells to reconstruct glial environments in the CNS. Brain Pathol 5: 443–450

Bottenstein J, Hayashi I, Hutchings S, Masui H, Mather J, McCLure DB, Ohasa S, Rizzino A, Sato G, Serrero G, Wolfe R, Wu R (1979) The growth of cells in serum-free hormone-supplemented media. Methods Enzymol 58: 94–109

Bonfanti L, Poulain DA, Theodosis DT (1993) Putative factors implicated in the structural plasticity of the hypothalamoneurohypophyseal system. Regul Pept 45: 165–170

Doucette JR (1984) The glial cells in the nerve fiber layer of the rat olfactory bulb. Anat Rec 210: 385–391

Farbman AI (1990) Olfactory neurogenesis: genetic or environmental controls? Trends Neurosci 13: 362–365

Franceschini IA, Barnett SC (1996) Low-affinity NGF-receptor and E-N-CAM expression define two types of olfactory nerve ensheathing cells that share a common lineage. Dev Biol 173: 327–343

Franklin RJM, Barnett SC (1997) Do olfactory glia have advantages over Schwann cells for CNS repair? J Neurosci Res 50: 1–8

Franklin RJM, Barnett SC (2000) Olfactory ensheathing cells and CNS regeneration: the sweet smell of success? Neuron 28: 1–4

Franklin RJ, Blakemore WF (1998) Transplanting myelin-forming cells into the central nervous system: principles and practice. Methods 16: 311–319

Franklin RJ, Gilson JM, Franceschini IA, Barnett SC (1996) Schwann cell-like myelination following transplantation of an olfactory bulb-ensheathing cell line into areas of demyelination in the adult CNS. Glia 17: 217–224

Imaizumi T, Lankford KL, Waxman SG, Greer CA, Kocsis JD (1998) Transplanted olfactory ensheathing cells remyelinate and enhance axonal conduction in the demyelinated dorsal columns of the rat spinal cord. J Neurosci 18: 6176–6185

Imaizumi T, Kato T, Honmou O, Uede T, Hashi K (2000) Transplantation of human olfactory ensheathing cells elicits remyelination of demyelinated rat spinal cord. Glia 30: 209–218

Li Y, Field PM, Raisman G (1997) Repair of adult rat corticospinal tract by transplants of olfactory ensheathing cells. Science 277: 2000–2002

Li Y, Field PM, Raisman G (1998) Regeneration of adult rat corticospinal axons induced by transplanted olfactory ensheathing cells. J Neurosci 18: 10514–10524

Lu J, Feron F, Ho SM, Mackay-Sim A, Waite PME (2001) Transplantation of nasal olfactory tissue promotes partial recovery in paraplegic adult rats. Brain Res 889: 344–357

Moran DT, Rowley JC, Jafek BW (1982) The fine structure of the human olfactory mucosa in man. J Neurocytol 11: 721–746

Morrison EE, Costanzo RM (1990) Morphology of the human olfactory epithelium. J Comp Neurol 297: 1–13

Muller F, O'Rahilly R (1990) The human brain at stages 21–23, with particular reference to the cerebral cortical plate and to the development of the cerebellum. Anat Embryol 182: 375–400

Nakashima T, Kimmelman CP, Snow JB (1984) Structure of human fetal and adult olfactory neuro-epithelium. Arch Otolaryngol 71: 49–62

Nakashima T, Kimmelman CP, Snow JB Jr (1985) Immunohistopathology of human olfactory epithelium, nerve and bulb. Laryngoscope 95: 391–396

Navarro X, Valero A, Gudino G, Fores J, Rodriguez FJ, Verdu E, Pascual R, Cuadras J, Nieto-Sampedre M (1999) Ensheathing glia transplants promote dorsal root regeneration and spinal reflex restitution after multiple lumbar rhizotomy. Ann Neurol 45: 207–215

Noble MD, Murray K (1984) Purified astrocytes promote the in vitro division of a bipotential glial progenitor cell. EMBO J 3: 2243–2247

Pixley SK (1992) The olfactory nerve contains two populations of glia, identified both in vivo and in vitro. Glia 5: 269–284

Pollock GS, Graham G, Marchionni MA, Barnett SC (1999) Neuregulin is a mitogen and survival factor for olfactory bulb ensheathing cell and is an isoform produced by astrocytes. Eur J Neurosci 11: 769–780

Raisman G (1985) Specialized neuroglial arrangement may explain the capacity of vomeronasal axons to reinnervate central neurons. Neuroscience 14: 237–254

Raisman G (2001) Olfactory ensheathing cells: another miracle cure for spinal cord injury. Nat Rev Neurosci 2: 369–374

Ramon-Cueto A, Nieto-Sampedro M (1992) Glial cells from adult rat olfactory bulb: immunocytochemical properties of pure cultures of ensheathing cells. Neuroscience 47: 213–220

Ramon-Cueto A, Nieto-Sampedro M (1994) Regeneration into the spinal cord of transected dorsal root axons is promoted by ensheathing glia transplants. Exp Neurol 127: 232–244

Ramon-Cueto A, Perez J, Nieto-Sampedro M (1993) In vitro enfolding of olfactory neurites by p75 NGF receptor positive ensheathing cells from adult rat olfactory bulb. Eur J Neurosci 5: 1172–11780

Ramon-Cueto A, Cordero MI, Santos-Benito FF, Avila J (2000) Functional recovery of paraplegic rats and motor axon regeneration in their spinal cords by olfactory ensheathing glia. Neuron 25: 425–435

Seki T, Rutishauser U (1998) Removal of polysialic acid neural cell adhesion molecule induces aberrant mossy fiber innervation and ectopic synaptogenesis in the hippocampus. J Neurosci 18: 3757–3766

Smale KA, Doucette R, Kawaja MD (1996) Implantation of olfactory ensheathing cells in the adult rat brain following fimbria-fornix transection. Exp Neurol 137: 225–233

Theodosis DT, Bonhomme R, Vitiello S, Rougon G, Poulain DA (1999) Cell surface expression of polysialic acid on NCAM is a prerequisite for activity-dependent morphological neuronal and glial plasticity. J Neurosci 19: 10228–10236

Yan H, Bunge MB, Wood PM, Plant GW (2001) Mitogenic response of adult rat olfactory ensheathing glia to four growth factors. Glia 33: 334–342

Advances in understanding and use of autoantibodies as markers of diseases

Marvin J. Fritzler* and **Leeanne J. Schoenroth**

Department of Medicine, University of Calgary, Calgary, Alberta, Canada

Introduction

Human autoantibodies have a significant place in the history of clinical and molecular medicine. First, dating to original observations of the LE cell in 1948 (Hargraves et al. 1948) to the present-day applications of array analyses, their use as diagnostic and prognostic markers of disease has been a valuable adjunct to clinical medicine (Tan 1991, 1999). Second, the role of autoantibodies in the pathogenesis of the disease has provided some useful approaches to therapy (G. Hahn 1986, B. Hahn et al. 2001). Third, a significant impact has been felt in the field of cell and molecular biology, where human autoantibodies have opened new fields of study and resulted in significant incremental knowledge through their use as reagents to discover and understand the function of novel cellular compartments (Tan 1991, von Muhlen and Tan 1995, Fritzler 1996). Small nuclear ribonucleoproteins (snRNPs) and the splicesome (Tan 1991, Lerner and Steitz 1981), unique centromere/kinetochore (Earnshaw and Rothfield 1985, Rattner 1995), nucleolar (Reimer et al. 1987, Fritzler 1993), Golgi complex (Chan and Fritzler 1998), and endosome (Selak et al. 1999, Waite et al. 1998) proteins were all elucidated through the use of human autoantibodies.

The spectrum of autoantibodies in autoimmune diseases, especially the systemic or non-organ-specific diseases, is constantly expanding. Autoantibodies to double-stranded DNA, histones, snRNPs (Sm, U1-RNP), and SS-A/Ro are commonly seen in systemic lupus erythematosus (SLE) (von Muhlen and Tan 1995) and the list of newer autoantibodies continues to expand (Table 1). Autoantibodies to centrosomes, the mitotic spindle apparatus, and components of the Golgi complex (referred to as golgins) provide unique reagents to study these cell organelles (Fig. 1). In addition, although many of these newer autoantibodies are rare, they

* Author's address: Department of Medicine, University of Calgary, 3330 Hospital Drive N.W., Calgary, AB, Canada T2N 4N1.
E-mail: fritzler@ucalgary.ca

Table 1. Newer autoantibodies described in systemic rheumatic diseases (partly extracted from von Muhlen et al. [1998])

Alpha fodrin	Collagen type II	Nuclear matrix
Annexin V	Early endosome antigen 1	Nuclear matrix and pore complex
Anti-sense ERCC1 (ASE1)	Fibronectin	p53
Apo A1	Golgins (Golgi complex)	Platelet membrane glycoproteins
Calreticulin	HSP90	Proteosome alpha-type subunit
CD4, CD45, CD36	Insulin receptor	Replication protein A
CENP-E	LSmD (like Sm D4)	RNA helicase
CENP-F	Nerve growth factor	Thyroglobulin

may hold diagnostic value. For example, approximately 50% of patients with antibodies to CENP-F (Fig. 1 E, F) have a malignancy (Casiano et al. 1995, Rattner et al. 1997). And, anti-golgin antibodies (Fig. 1 G, H) are most commonly associated with Sjögren's syndrome sera that may not contain other classical serological markers such as anti-SS-A/Ro antibodies.

Origin of autoantibodies: mutations and xenobiotics

The origin of autoantibodies is unknown and numerous theories have been proposed. Those in vogue today include an inherent dysregulation of the immune system, molecular mimicry, and antigens that are altered by mutations from exposure to drugs or toxins (Fritzler and Salazar 1991, Fritzler 1997). The appearance of some autoantibodies may point to inciting agents such as viruses and up-regulated proteins produced during cell proliferation and cell death or to antigens altered by mutagenesis (Imai et al. 1993a, b; Fritzler 1997; Fritzler and Salazar 1991; Mountz et al. 1994). One of the fastest growing fields in autoimmunity is the study of autoantibodies in cancer (Imai et al. 1992, 1995; Ochs et al. 1994; Mudenda et al. 1994; Overwijk and Restifo 2001), where evidence that gene mutations of antigens may lead to the production of autoantibodies is supported by studies of p53 (Baron et al. 1982, Dalifard et al. 1999). It is known that p53 can be highly mutated in cancer cells and is a target autoantigen in these and other conditions (Soussi 2000, Mudenda et al. 1994, Lubin et al. 1993, Kovacs et al. 1997, Herkel et al. 2000). This knowledge would suggest the hypothesis that the mutated protein would be recognized as foreign and that in response, antibodies would be generated to the mutated epitope on p53. Surprisingly, the epitopes on p53 bound by autoantibodies found in cancer patients do not bind to the hypermutated domain of the protein but primarily bind to the "normal" or unmutated domains (Soussi 2000).

Studies in the field of xenobiotic-induced autoimmunity and environmental toxicology are also starting to reveal interesting associations (Yang et al. 2001, Pollard et al. 2001, Bigazzi 1997). Xenobiotics are foreign substances of synthetic, natural, or biological origin and may include plant or animal products, industrial chemicals, and intentional or inadvertent exposure to drugs. There is evidence that aromatic hydrocarbons, carbamates, heavy metals, organophosphates, ozone,

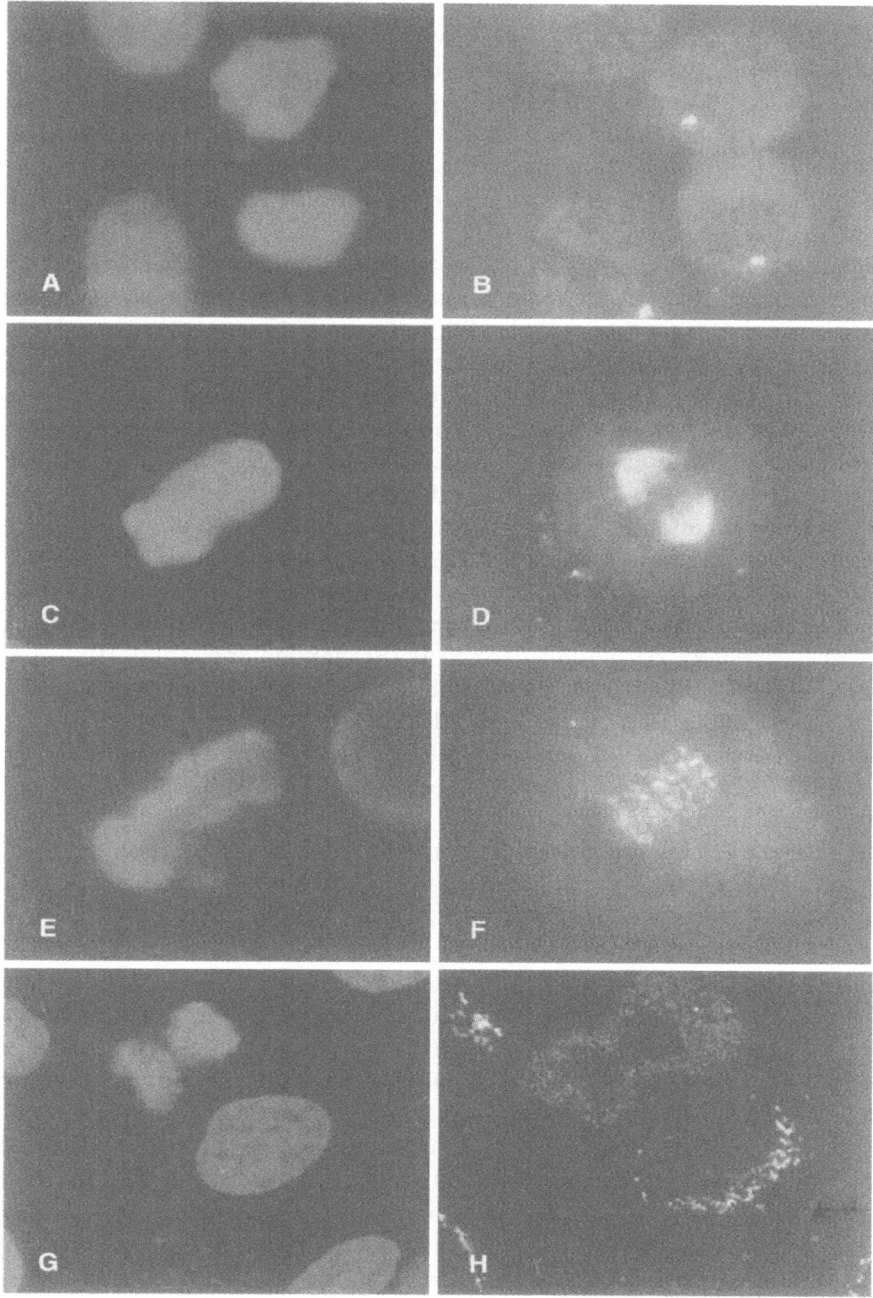

Fig. 1A–H. Indirect immunofluorescence of newer autoantibodies. HEp-2 cells were stained with human sera with antibodies to centrosomes (**A** and **B**), the mitotic spindle apparatus (**C** and **D**), centromere F (CENP-F) (**E** and **F**), and the Golgi apparatus (golgin-97) (**G** and **H**). Cells in panels A, C, E, and G have been stained with 4′,6-diamidino-2-phenylindole to show the location of cells, nuclei and metaphase chromatin. The same cells shown in panels B, D, F, and H are stained with human antibodies. Original magnification, ×400

nitrogen dioxide, polycyclic aromatic hydrocarbons, diethylstilbestrol, dioxin, and polychlorinated biphenyls affect the developing immune system (Barnett 1996). The relationship between several drugs and the induction of a lupus-like syndrome has been described, but the effects of exposure to environmental agents and their induction or autoantibodies are less well understood (Fritzler and Rubin 1993, Kavlock et al. 1996). The long-term effects of chronic exposure to xenobiotics or combinations of these agents on human health and genes are not well studied (Barnett 1996).

One exception is the study of antibodies to U3-RNP (fibrillarin) that are seen in approximately 15% of systemic sclerosis patients (Fritzler 1993, Arnett et al. 1996, Rothfield 1992, Okano et al. 1992). These autoantibodies are also seen in mice exposed to mercury, silver, and other heavy metals (Takeuchi et al. 1995; Hultman et al. 1989, 1994a, b; Füllekrug et al. 1999). Of relevance to these studies, a recently published study of a small cohort of systemic-sclerosis (SSc) patients showed that the patients with high-titer antibodies to fibrillarin had elevated levels of urinary mercury (Arnett et al. 2000).

More recently, attention is shifting to other environmental agents that bind to hormonal receptors or alter hormonal function. Among those of relevance to auto-immune diseases are molecules referred to as estrogen disruptors (Kavlock et al. 1996). The role of reproductive hormones in modulating autoimmune disease has long been suspected, particularly for SLE (Fernandes and Talal 1986, Golsteyn and Fritzler 1987, Blank et al. 1990, Lahita 1992). Pregnancy has been reported to be associated with an increased rate of flare in SLE (Petri et al. 1991) and there are reports of abnormal estrogen metabolism in SLE patients and family members (Lahita 1992). "Endocrine-disrupting chemicals (EDC)" or "endocrine disruptors" is a broad term including any exogenous agent that interferes with the production, release, transport, metabolism, binding, action, or elimination of natural hormones in the body responsible for the maintenance of homeostasis and the regulation of developmental processes (Kavlock et al. 1996). These may act via the estrogen receptor or by other mechanisms.

Estrogen has been shown to induce autoantibodies in normal mice (Verthelyi and Ahmed 1999) and enhance autoantibody expression in murine autoimmune models (B. Hahn 2001). Substances that have estrogenic activity can be broadly divided into "natural" and "synthetic" categories. Natural estrogens include those that are produced endogenously, such as phytoestrogens produced by plants and mycoestrogens by fungi. Phytoestrogens can be subdivided into three main classes: isoflavones, coumestans, and lignans. Soybeans and soy foods are the most significant dietary sources of isoflavones. Coumestrol and 4'-methoxy-coumestrol are found in alfalfa, clover, and other fodder crops. Lignans are found in flax seed and other oil seeds. Synthetic estrogens in the form of drugs and chemicals have been inadvertently or purposefully introduced into the ecosystem and, as a group, they are known as xenoestrogens. Xenoestrogens include pesticides such as 1,1,1-trichloro-2,2-bis(p-chlorophenyl) ethane (DDT), methoxychlor, dieldrin, and kepone; preservatives such as butylated hydroxyanisole; solvents including hydrocarbons; plasticizers such as bisphenol A and polychlorinated biphenyls.

Adverse health effects from EDCs have been identified primarily in wildlife species after relatively high exposure to xenoestrogens in the form of organochlorines (i.e., DDT and its metabolites), polychlorinated biphenyls, and dioxins, and to naturally occurring plant estrogens (Kavlock et al. 1996). Knowledge of the effects of EDCs in humans is largely limited to diethylstilbestrol. This is a synthetic estrogenic compound that is more potent than endogenous 17β-estradiol and was given to pregnant women to prevent miscarriage. It has been shown to produce reproductive tract abnormalities in men and women and vaginal clear cell adenocarcinoma in women exposed in utero (Golden et al. 1998). There has been reported an association between ingestion of alfalfa seeds and sprouts and the induction of a lupus-like syndrome including hemolytic anemia and high-titer anti-nuclear and anti-double-stranded DNA antibodies in primates (Montanaro and Bardana 1991). It is clear that with increased awareness of EDCs and xenoestrogens, it will be important to know how these substances influence autoantibody induction and disease expression.

Autoimmunity and biological therapeutics

In recent years, a great deal of interest has been generated with the introduction of chimeric antibodies directed to tumor necrosis factor (TNF) as effective agents in the treatment of rheumatoid arthritis, Crohn's disease, psoriasis, ankylosing spondylitis and juvenile arthritis (Bondeson and Maini 2001; Kalden 2000; D'Haens 1999, 2000; Mease et al. 2000; Gorman et al. 2001; Stone et al. 2001; Cavagna et al. 2001; Lovell et al. 2000). Despite the apparent efficacy of this treatment modality, anecdotal reports suggest that patients treated with TNF-blocking agents can develop anti-double-stranded DNA and other features of SLE and related conditions (Pisetsky 2000, Charles et al. 2000, Saleem et al. 2001). This is interesting in light of historical observations that certain drugs also induce a lupus-like syndrome accompanied by high titers of autoantibodies to nucleosomes (Fritzler and Rubin 1993, Burlingame and Rubin 1996, Rubin and Burlingame 1991, Mongey and Hess 1993). Therefore, postmarketing surveillance becomes an important consideration for physicians that adopt newer therapeutic strategies for autoimmune diseases and patients on these protocols may need to be monitored for the appearance of autoantibodies and drug-induced disease.

Pathogenic role of autoantibodies

A question that arises from the study of autoantibodies in the sera of patients with systemic rheumatic diseases is whether these antibodies participate in the disease processes. Unlike a clearer role for autoantibodies to the acetylcholine receptor in myasthenia gravis or parietal cell antibodies in pernicious anemia (Drachman et al. 1982, Gomez and Richman 1983, Bigazzi et al. 1992), it has been difficult to understand how antibodies directed against intracellular components are involved in the pathogenesis. The relevance of observations that autoantibodies gain entry into living cells (Alarcon-Segovia et al. 1978, 1979, 1996a, b) is still controversial.

Table 2. Autoantibodies demonstrating inhibition of cellular function (von Muhlen and Tan 1995)[a]

Autoantibody	Function inhibited
tRNA synthetases	Charging tRNAs with amino acids
CENP-B	Moving chromosomes at metaphase
PCNA	Replicating DNA strands
Ribosome P proteins	Translating mRNA
Pyruvate dehydrogenase E2	Binding lipoic acid to mitochondrial enzymes
Sm/U1RNP	Splicing precursor mRNA
DNA topoisomerase I	Altering DNA topology
RNA polymerase I	Synthesizing 18S and 28S RNA
RNA polymerase II	Transcribing mRNA
RNA polymerase III	Synthesizing 5S rRNA and tRNA

[a] CENP, centromere protein; mRNA, messenger RNA; PCNA, proliferating cell nuclear antigen; RNP, ribonucleoprotein; rRNA, ribosomal RNA; tRNA, transfer RNA

Some of the best evidence for a pathogenic role of autoantibodies directed against intracellular antigens comes from studies of anti-chromatin and anti-SS-A/Ro antibodies. Antibodies directed against chromatin components have been shown in animal models and humans to participate in the pathogenesis of renal disease (for reviews see Stollar 1990, van Bruggen et al. 1994). Although this might be seen as a rather passive role in the disease processes, other evidence indicates that some autoantibodies bind to and inhibit the functional or physiological role of intracellular antigens (Bachman et al. 1990, Leung and Gershwin 1990, Tan 1989, von Muhlen and Tan 1995) (Table 2). Although the significance of these observations in the pathophysiology of systemic rheumatic diseases remains to be elucidated, it seems unlikely that these antibodies exert a pathogenic effect through inhibition of intracellular protein or enzyme function in vivo.

Studies of the SS-A/Ro autoantigen system have also provided some insight into the pathogenic role of autoantibodies in a subset of SLE patients. Antibodies to SS-A/Ro were first found in high frequency in patients with primary Sjögren's syndrome and SLE and in lower frequency in other rheumatic diseases (von Muhlen and Tan 1995, Tan 1999, Chan and Buyon 1994). A pathogenic role for anti-SS-A/Ro in the production of the cutaneous and cardiac lesions of the neonatal lupus syndrome has been suggested by the observation that, as the cutaneous lesions resolve, maternally derived SS-A/Ro disappears from the infant's circulation (Buyon et al. 1994, Tseng and Buyon 1997). This has been supported by biochemical evidence showing that these antibodies or their genes are highly expressed in diseased hearts and skin, and these autoantibodies can produce physiological changes compatible with their presumed pathogenic role in the fetus (Buyon et al. 1997, Miranda-Carús et al. 2000, Miranda et al. 1998, Tseng et al. 1996).

Advances in diagnostics

Over 50 year ago Hargraves first described the LE cell (Hargraves et al. 1948) and this was followed several years later by the adoption of indirect immuno-fluorescence (IIF) techniques (Fritzler 1986, Harmon et al. 1984, Xia et al. 1987). In retrospect, it is interesting that these techniques had an astonishing life-span. LE cell preparations are still performed in a few laboratories and IIF remains a screening test of choice despite advances in the use of immunodiffusion (Clark et al. 1969, Takano et al. 1989), counterimmunoelectrophoresis (Manoussakis et al. 1993, Meilof et al. 1990, Bossuyt et al. 2000), immunoblotting (Ben-Chetrit et al. 1988, Rader et al. 1989, Buyon et al. 1990, Slobbe et al. 1991), immunoprecipitation (Wolin and Steitz 1984, Forman et al. 1985), and enzyme-linked immunosorbent assay (ELISA) (Manoussakis et al. 1993, Meilof et al. 1990). It has been recognized that most of these techniques have limitations in a clinical laboratory. For example, immunodiffusion lacks sensitivity and can take up to 48 h before precipitin lines are visible or interpretable. Immunoblotting is expensive and time consuming, and not all autoantibodies are detected by this technique (Boire and Craft 1990, Boire et al. 1991). Counterimmunoelectrophoresis is useful to detect high-titer antibodies but may not discriminate between reactivity of sera with antibodies to certain antigens that are part of the same macromolecular complex (Manoussakis et al. 1993, Meilof et al. 1990). Immunoprecipitation protocols that use extracts from radiolabeled cells are not suitable for the clinical detection of some autoanti-bodies because many sera are negative in this assay (Chan and Buyon 1994). ELISA techniques are the protocol of choice for clinical laboratories that rely on high volume and rapid reporting of results. Unfortunately, it appears that stand-ardization of these assays has not been achieved since discrepant results were produced in different laboratories using a number of commercial kits (Tan et al. 2002). ELISA using recombinant antigens can be a highly specific and sensitive assay for SS-A/Ro protein, but it is expensive and has not been validated in mul-ticenter trials. Recently, natural and recombinant antigens have been placed in discrete lines on strips of a solid-phase backing that allow convenient detection of autoantibodies by modified immunoblotting techniques (Bossuyt et al. 2000).

A more recent approach to improve the sensitivity and specificity of assays that detect SS-A/Ro antibodies is to employ the technique of transfection where the appropriate gene(s) are inserted into cells. This technique introduces multiple copies of the gene that under the control of specific promoter-regulator genes leads to stable "overexpression" of the gene of interest. This approach has been utilized in the development of an IIF substrate that utilizes HEp-2 cells transfected with a full-length human 60 kDa SS-A/Ro cDNA (Keech et al. 1994, Fritzler and Miller 1995). Since its introduction, a number of clinical laboratories have evalu-ated this commercially available substrate and reported relatively high sensitivity and specificity for the detection of SS-A/Ro antibodies (Fritzler and Miller 1995, Keech et al. 1996, Pollock and Toh 1999, Bossuyt et al. 2000, Morozzi et al. 2000, Peene et al. 2000).

The advent of genomics, ribonomics, and proteomics is moving newer protein array technologies to the forefront. These technologies include autoantigens that

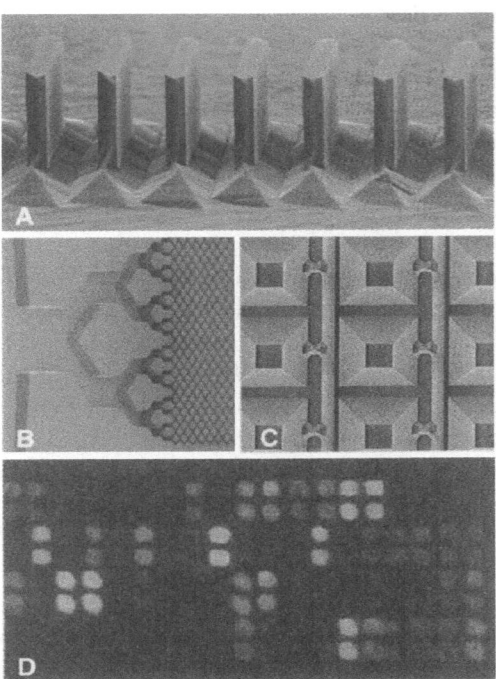

Fig. 2A–D. A theoretical approach to antigen array testing with a biochip array. A single drop of blood is applied to the chip and a comb at the entry point (**A**) removes the blood cells permitting the plasma to flow down a series of channels (**B**) to come in contact with the antigens that have been spotted on a flat surface (**C**). After appropriate incubation and reaction with a secondary antibody conjugated with a fluorochrome, the reactivity with the antigens on each surface is visualized as a fluorescent signal (**D**)

are bound on an appropriate solid-phase matrix or are bound to beads impregnated with a spectrum of laser-reactive fluorochromes. Protein arrays offer advantages of rapid results and the potential to identify a broader pattern of autoantibodies in a single serum. Some of the conceptual aspects of this technology are shown in Fig. 2. Theoretically, a single drop of blood can be applied to the chip and a comb at the application site (Fig. 2A) retards blood cells and prevents them from flowing forward. The plasma is evenly distributed along channels (Fig. 2B) to the arrays of autoantigens that are spotted on the chip (Fig. 2C). After appropriate incubation, washing away excess antibody, and the application of a fluorochrome-labeled secondary antibody, the reactivity with autoantigens is detected fluorometrically and the reactivity displayed as a fluorescent "map" (Fig. 2D).

In the future, new approaches that employ nanotechnology and microfluidics are likely to find a niche in diagnostics as well (Moore 2001, Mitchell 2001, Davies 2001, Woolley 2001, Stokes et al. 2001). Nanotechnology is an engineering discipline with the goal of building structures that have every atom in the proper place. With this technology it will be possible to build and replicate almost any covalently bonded structure and identical molecules will truly be identical. These features will alleviate some of the challenges of reproducibility confronting many

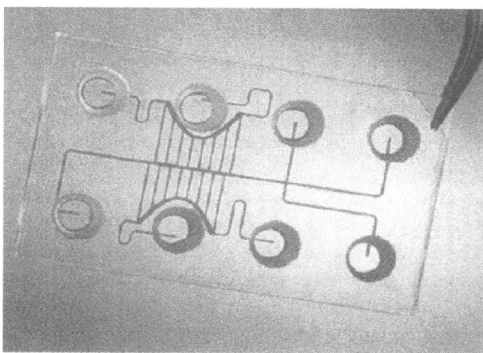

Fig. 3. Example of a biochip that is manufactured for microfluidics applications. Serum, antigens, diluents, and analytes would be placed in one of the appropriate wells (shown as circles) and the reactivity of antibody with antigen monitored by changes in physico-chemical or electrochemical properties

diagnostic platforms today. Microfluidics can use a variety of approaches such as a 2-dimensional photosensor array biochip that contains a serum or antibody delivery system, an antigen delivery system, a reagent delivery system, and other components (see Fig. 3). One advantage of these systems is that both quantitative and qualitative results are known within seconds. As research progresses in this area it may be possible to simplify the approach such that only the antigen and the antibody delivery systems are required with the resulting antigen-antibody complex being detected as a unique physico-chemical structure.

References

Alarcon-Segovia D, Ruiz-Arguelles A, Fishbein E (1978) Antibody to nuclear ribonucleoprotein penetrates live human mononuclear cells through Fc receptors. Nature 271: 67–69

Alarcon-Segovia D, Ruiz-Arguelles A, Fishbein E (1979) Antibody penetration into living cells I: intranuclear immunoglobulin in peripheral blood mononuclear cells in mixed connective tissue disease and systemic lupus erythematosus. Clin Exp Immunol 35: 364–375

Alarcon-Segovia D, Llorente L, Ruiz-Arguelles A (1996a) Autoantibodies that penetrate into living cells. In: Peter JB, Shoenfeld Y (eds) Autoantibodies. Elsevier, Amsterdam, pp 96–102

Alarcon-Segovia D, Ruiz-Arguelles A, Llorente L (1996b) Broken dogma: penetration of autoantibodies into living cells. Immunol Today 17: 163–164

Arnett FC, Reveille JD, Goldstein R, Pollard KM, Leaird K, Smith EA, Carwile EC, Fritzler MJ (1996) Autoantibodies to fibrillarin in systemic sclerosis (scleroderma): an immunogenetic, serological and clinical analysis. Arthritis Rheum 39: 1151–1160

Arnett FC, Fritzler MJ, Ahn C, Holian A (2000) Urinary mercury levels in patients with autoantibodies to U3-RNP (fibrillarin). J Rheumatol 27: 405–410

Bachman M, Pfeifer K, Schroder HC, Muller WEG (1990) Characterization of the autoantigen La as a nucleic acid-dependent ATPase/dATPase with melting properties. Cell 60: 85–93

Barnett J (1996) Statement from the work session on chemically-induced alterations in the developing immune system: the wildlife/human connection. Environ Health Perspect 104: 807–808

Baron M, Lee P, Keystone EC (1982) The articular manifestations of progressive systemic sclerosis (scleroderma). Ann Rheum Dis 41: 147–152

Ben-Chetrit E, Chan EKL, Sullivan KF, Tan EM (1988) A 52-kD protein is a novel component of the SS-A/Ro antigenic particle. J Exp Med 167: 1560–1571

Bigazzi PE (1997) Autoimmunity caused by xenobiotics. Toxicology 119: 1–21

Bigazzi PE, Burek CL, Rose NR (1992) Antibodies to tissue-specific endocrine, gastrointestinal, and surface-receptor antigens. In: Rose NR, de Macario EC, Fahey JL, Friedman H, Penn GM (eds) Manual of clinical laboratory immunology. American Society for Microbiology, Washington, DC, pp 765–774

Blank M, Mendlovic S, Fricke H, Mozes E, Talal N, Shoenfeld Y (1990) Sex hormone involvement in the induction of experimental systemic lupus erythematosus by a pathogenic anti-DNA idiotype in naive mice. J Rheumatol 17: 311–317

Boire G, Craft J (1990) Human Ro ribonucleoprotein particles: characterization of native structure and stable association with the La polypeptide. J Clin Invest 85: 1182–1190

Boire G, Lopez-Longo F-J, Lapointe S, Menard H-A (1991) Sera from patients with autoimmune disease recognize conformational determinants on the 60-kd Ro/SS-A protein. Arthritis Rheum 34: 722–729

Bondeson J, Maini RN (2001) Tumour necrosis factor as a therapeutic target in rheumatoid arthritis and other chronic inflammatory diseases: the clinical experience with infliximab (Remicade). Int J Clin Pract 55: 211–216

Bossuyt X, Meurs L, Mewis A, Marien G, Blanckaert N (2000) Screening for autoantibodies to SS-A/Ro by indirect immunofluorescence using HEp-2000TM cells. Ann Clin Biochem 37: 216–219

Burlingame RW, Rubin RL (1996) Autoantibody to the nucleosome subunit (H2A-H2B)-DNA is an early and ubiquitous feature of lupus-like conditions. Mol Biol Rep 23: 159–166

Buyon JP, Slade SG, Chan EKL, Tan EM, Winchester R (1990) Effective separation of the 52 kDa SSA/Ro polypeptide from the 48 kDa SSB/La polypeptide by altering conditions of polyacrylamide gel electrophoresis. J Immunol Methods 129: 207–210

Buyon JP, Waltuck J, Caldwell K, Crawford B, Slade SG, Copel J, Chan EKL (1994) Relationship between maternal and neonatal levels of antibodies to 48 kDa SSB(La), 52 kDa SSA(Ro), and 60 kDa SSA(Ro) in pregnancies complicated by congenital heart block. J Rheumatol 21: 1943–1950

Buyon JP, Tseng CE, DiDonato F, Rashbaum W, Morris A, Chan EKL (1997) Cardiac expression of 52β, an alternative transcript of the congenital heart block-associated 52-kd SS-A/Ro autoantigen, is maximal during fetal development. Arthritis Rheum 40: 655–660

Casiano CA, Humbel RL, Peebles C, Covini G, Tan EM (1995) Autoimmunity to the cell cycle-dependent centromere protein p330$^{d/CENP-F}$ in disorders associated with cell proliferation. J Autoimmun 8: 575–586

Cavagna L, Caporali R, Epis O, Bobbio-Pallavicini F, Montecucco C (2001) Inflixamab in the treatment of adult Still's disease refractory to conventional therapy. Clin Exp Rheumatol 19: 329–332

Chan EKL, Buyon JP (1994) The SS-A/Ro antigen. In: Van Venrooij W, Maini RN (eds) Manual of biological markers of disease. Kluwer, Dordrecht, pp 1–18

Chan EKL, Fritzler MJ (1998) Golgins: coiled-coil-rich proteins associated with the Golgi complex. Electronic J Biotechnol 1: http://ejb.ucv.cl/content/vol1/issue2/full/1

Charles PJ, Smeenk RJT, DeJong J, Feldman M, Maini RN (2000) Assessment of antibodies to double-stranded DNA induced in rheumatoid arthritis patients following treatment with imflixamab, a monoclonal antibody to tumor necrosis factor α. Arthritis Rheum 43: 2383–2390

Clark G, Reichlin M, Tomasi TB (1969) Characterization of a soluble cytoplasmic antigen reactive with sera from patients with systemic lupus erythematosus. J Immunol 102: 117–122

Dalifard I, Daver A, Larra F (1999) Cytosolic p53 protein and serum p53 autoantibody evaluation in breast cancer: comparison with prognostic factors. Anticancer Res 19: 5015–5022

Davies MJ (2001) Microfluidics venture. Trends Biotechnol 19: 331–332

D'Haens GR (1999) Infliximab (Remicade), a new biological treatment for Crohn's disease. Ital J Gastroenterol Hepatol 31: 519–520

D'Haens G (2000) Infliximab (Remicade): the magic bullet for Crohn's disease? Dig Liver Dis 32: 653–656

Drachman DB, Adams RN, Josifek LF, Self SG (1982) Functional activities of autoantibodies to acetylcholine receptors and the clinical severity of myasthenia gravis. N Engl J Med 307: 769–775

Earnshaw WC, Rothfield N (1985) Identification of a family of human centromere proteins using autoimmune sera from patients with scleroderma. Chromosoma 91: 313–321

Fernandes G, Talal N (1986) SLE: hormones and diet. Clin Exp Rheumatol 4: 183–185

Forman MS, Nakamura M, Mimori T, Gelpi C, Hardin JA (1985) Detection of antibodies to small nuclear ribonucleoproteins and small cytoplasmic ribonucleoproteins using unlabeled cell extracts. Arthritis Rheum 28: 1356–1361

Fritzler MJ (1986) Autoantibody testing: procedures and significance in systemic rheumatic diseases. Methods Achiev Exp Pathol 12: 224–260

Fritzler MJ (1993) Autoantibodies in scleroderma. J Dermatol 20: 257–268

Fritzler MJ (1996) Clinical relevance of autoantibodies in systemic rheumatic diseases. Mol Biol Rep 23: 133–145

Fritzler MJ (1997) Autoantibodies: diagnostic fingerprints and etiologic perplexities. Clin Invest Med 20: 50–66

Fritzler MJ, Miller BJ (1995) Detection of autoantibodies to SS-A/Ro by indirect immunofluorescence using a transfected and overexpressed human 60 kD Ro autoantigen in HEp-2 cells. J Clin Lab Anal 9: 218–224

Fritzler MJ, Rubin RL (1993) Drug-induced lupus. In: Dubois EL, Hahn B, Wallace DJ (eds) Dubois' lupus erythematosus. Lea & Febiger, Philadelphia, pp 442–453

Fritzler MJ, Salazar M (1991) The diversity and origin of rheumatologic autoantibodies. Clin Microbiol Rev 4: 256–269

Füllekrug J, Scheiffele P, Simons K (1999) VIP36 localisation to the early secretory pathway. J Cell Sci 112: 2813–2821

Golden RJ, Noller KL, Titus-Ernstoff L, Kaufman RH, Mittendorf R, Stillman R, Reese EA (1998) Environmental endocrine modulators and human health: an assessment of the biological evidence. Crit Rev Toxicol 28: 109–227

Golsteyn EJ, Fritzler MJ (1987) Review: The role of the thymus-hypothalamus-pituitary-gonadal axis in normal immun processes and autoimmunity. J Rheumatol 14: 982–990

Gomez CM, Richman DP (1983) Anti-acetylcholine receptor antibodies directed against the α-bungarotoxin binding site induce a unique form of experimental myasthenia. Proc Natl Acad Sci USA 80: 4089–4093

Gorman JD, Sack KE, Davis JC (2001) A randomized, double-blind, placebo-controlled trial of etanercept (Enbrel®) in the treatment of ankylosing spondylitis. Arthritis Rheum 44: S91

Hahn BH (2001) Animal models of systemic lupus erythematosus. In: Wallace DJ, Hahn BH (eds) Dubois' lupus erythematosus. Lippincott Williams & Wilkins, Philadelphia, pp 339–388

Hahn BH, Singh RR, Wong WK, Tsao BP, Bulpitt K, Ebling FM (2001) Treatment with a consensus peptide based on amino acid sequences in autoantibodies prevents T cell activation by autoantigens and delays disease onset in murine lupus. Arthritis Rheum 44: 432–441

Hahn GS (1986) Immunoglobulin-derived drugs. Nature 324: 283–284

Hargraves MM, Richmond H, Morton R (1948) Presentation of two bone marrow elements: the "tart" cells and the "L.E." cell. Mayo Clin Proc 27: 25–28

Harmon CE, Deng JS, Peebles CL, Tan EM (1984) The importance of tissue substrate in the SS-ARo antigen-antibody system. Arthritis Rheum 27: 166–173

Herkel J, Erez-Alon N, Mimran A, Wolkowicz R, Harmelin A, Ruiz P, Rotter V, Cohen IR (2000) Systemic lupus erythematosus in mice, spontaneous and induced, is associated with autoimmunity to the C-terminal domain of p53 that recognizes damaged DNA. Eur J Immunol 30: 977–984

Hultman P, Enestrom S, Pollard KM, Tan EM (1989) Anti-fibrillarin antibodies in mercury-treated mice. Clin Exp Immunol 78: 470–472

Hultman P, Enestrom S, Turley SJ, Pollard KM (1994a) Selective induction of anti-fibrillarin autoantibodies by silver nitrate in mice. Clin Exp Immunol 96: 285–291

Hultman P, Johansson U, Turley SJ, Lindh U, Eneström S, Pollard KM (1994b) Adverse immunological effects and autoimmunity induced by dental amalgam and alloy in mice. FASEB J 8: 1183–1190

Imai H, Ochs RL, Kiyosawa K, Furuta S, Nakamura RM, Tan EM (1992) Nucleolar antigens and auto-antibodies in hepatocellular carcinoma and other malignancies. Am J Pathol 140: 859–870

Imai H, Chan EKL, Kiyosawa K, Fu XD, Tan EM (1993a) Novel nuclear autoantigen with splicing factor motifs identified with antibody from hepatocellular carcinoma. J Clin Invest 92: 2419–2426

Imai H, Nakano Y, Kiyosawa K, Tan EM (1993b) Increasing titers and changing specificities of anti-nuclear antibodies in patients with chronic liver disease who develop hepatocellular carcinoma. Cancer 71: 26–35

Imai H, Furuta K, Landberg G, Kiyosawa K, Liu LF, Tan EM (1995) Autoantibody to DNA topoisomerase II in primary liver cancer. Clin Cancer Research 1: 417–424

Kalden JR (2000) The application of infliximab (Remicade), a chimeric monoclonal antibody, in the treatment of rheumatic diseases. Isr Med Assoc J 2 Suppl: 11-2-1-12

Kavlock RJ, Daston GP, DeRosa C, Fenner-Crisp P, Gray LE, Kaattari S, Lucier G, Luster M, Mac MJ, Maczka C, Miller R, Moore J, Rolland R, Scott GSDM, Sinks T, Tilson HA (1996) Research needs for the risk assessment of health and environmental effects of endocrine disruptors: a report of the U.S. EPA-sponsored Workshop. Environ Health Perspect 104: 715–808

Keech CL, McCluskey J, Gordon TP (1994) Transfection and overexpression of the human 60-kDa Ro/SS-A autoantigen in HEp-2 cells. Clin Immunol Immunopathol 73: 146–151

Keech CL, Howarth S, Coates T, Rischmueller M, McCluskey J, Gordon TP (1996) Rapid and sensitive detection of anti-Ro (SS-A) antibodies by indirect immunofluorescence of 60 kDa Ro HEp-2 transfectants. Pathology 28: 54–57

Kovacs B, Patel A, Hershey JN, Dennis GJ, Kirschfink M, Tsokos GC (1997) Antibodies against p53 in sera from patients with systemic lupus erythematosus and other rheumatic diseases. Arthritis Rheum 40: 980–985

Lahita RG (1992) The importance of estrogens in systemic lupus erythematosus. Clin Immunol Immunopathol 63: 17–18

Lerner MR, Steitz JA (1981) Snurps and scyrps. Cell 25: 298–300

Leung PSC, Gershwin ME (1990) The molecular structure of autoantigens. Curr Opin Immunol 2: 567–575

Lovell DJ, Giannini EH, Reiff A, Cawkwell GD, Silverman ED, Nocton JJ (2000) Etanercept in children with polyarticular juvenile rheumatoid arthritis. N Engl J Med 342: 763–769

Lubin R, Schlichtholz B, Bengoufa D, Zalcman G, Tredaniel J, Hirsch A, Caron de Fromentel C, Preudhomme C, Fenaux P, Fournier G, Mangin P, Laurent-Puig P, Pelletier G, Schlumberger M, Desgrandchamps F, Le Duc A, Peyrat JP, Janin N, Bressac B, Soussi T (1993) Analysis of p53 antibodies in patients with various cancers define B-cell epitopes of human p53: distribution on primary structure and exposure on protein surface. Cancer Res 53: 5872–5876

Manoussakis MN, Kistis KG, Liu X, Aidinis V, Guialis A, Moutsopoulos HM (1993) Detection of anti-Ro(SS-A) antibodies in autoimmune diseases: comparison of five methods. Br J Rheumatol 32: 449–455

Mease PJ, Goffe MS, Metz J, VanderStoep A, Finck B, Burge DJ (2000) Etanercept in the treatment of psoraitic arthritis and psoriasis: a randomized trial. Lancet 356: 385–390

Meilof JF, Bantjes I, de Jong J, Van Dam AP, Smeenk RJT (1990) The detection of anti-Ro(SS-A) and anti-La(SS-B) antibodies: a comparison of counterimmunoelectrophoresis with immunoblot, ELISA, and RNA-precipitation assays. J Immunol Methods 133: 215–226

Miranda ME, Tseng CE, Rashbaum W, Ochs RL, Casiano CA, Di Donato F, Chan EKL, Buyon JP (1998) Accessibility of SSA/Ro and SSB/La antigens to maternal autoantibodies in apoptotic human fetal cardiac myocytes. J Immunol 161: 5061–5069

Miranda-Carús ME, Askanase AD, Clancy RM, Di Donato F, Chou TM, Libera MR, Chan EKL, Buyon JP (2000) Anti-SSA/Ro and anti-SSB/La autoantibodies bind the surface of apoptotic fetal cardiocytes and promote secretion of TNF-α by macrophages. J Immunol 165: 5345–5351

Mitchell P (2001) Microfluidics: downsizing large-scale biology. Nat Biotechnol 19: 717–721

Mongey AB, Hess EV (1993) Drug and environmental effects on the induction of autoimmunity. J Lab Clin Med 122: 652–657

Montanaro A, Bardana EJ (1991) Dietary amino acid-induced systemic lupus erythematosus. Rheum Dis Clin North Am 17: 323–332

Moore A (2001) Brave small world: biotechnology and nanotechnology may give rise to a completely new industry. EMBO Rep 2: 86–88

Morozzi G, Bellisai F, Simpatico A, Pucci G, Bacarelli MR, Campanella V, Marcolongo R, Galeazzi M (2000) Comparison of differrent methods for the detection of anti-Ro/SSAm antibodies in connective tissue diseases. Clin Exp Rheumatol 18: 729–731

Mountz JD, Wu J, Cheng J, Zhou T (1994) Autoimmune disease: a problem of defective apoptosis. Arthritis Rheum 37: 1415–1420

Mudenda B, Green JA, Green B, Jenkins JR, Robertson L, Tarunina M, Leinster SJ (1994) The relationship between serum p53 autoantibodies and characteristics of human breast cancer. Br J Cancer 69: 1115–1119

Ochs RL, Stein TW Jr, Tan EM (1994) Coiled bodies in the nucleolus of breast cancer cells. J Cell Sci 107: 385–399

Okano Y, Steen VD, Medsger TA Jr (1992) Autoantibody to U3 nucleolar ribonucleoprotein (fibrillarin) in patients with systemic sclerosis. Arthritis Rheum 35: 95–100

Overwijk WW, Restifo NP (2001) Autoimmunity and immunotherapy of cancer: targeting the "self" to destroy the "other". Crit Rev Immunol 20: 433–450

Peene I, Van Ael W, Vandenbossche M, Vervaet T, Veys E, De Keyser F (2000) Sensitivity of the HEp-2000 substrate for the detection of anti-SSA/Ro60 antibodies. Clin Rheumatol 19: 291–295

Petri M, Howard D, Repke J (1991) Frequency of lupus flare in pregnancy: the Hopkins lupus pregnancy center experience. Arthritis Rheum 34: 1538

Pisetsky DS (2000) Tumor necrosis factor alpha blockers and the induction of anti-DNA autoantibodies. Arthritis Rheum 43: 2381–2382

Pollard KM, Pearson DL, Hultman P, Deane TN, Lindh U, Kono DH (2001) Xenobiotic acceleration of idiopathic systemic autoimmunity in lupus-prone BXSB Mice. Environ Health Perspect 109: 27–33

Pollock W, Toh BH (1999) Routine immunofluorescence detection of Ro/SS-A autoantibody using HEp-2 cells transfected with human 60 kDa Ro/SS-A. J Clin Pathol 52: 684–687

Rader MD, O'Brien C, Liu Y, Harley JB, Reichlin M (1989) Heterogeneity of the Ro/SSA antigen: different molecular forms in lymphocytes and red blood cells. J Clin Invest 83: 1293–1298

Rattner JB (1995) Centromeres and telomeres. In: Bittar EE, Bittar N (eds) Principles of medical biology. JAI Press, Greenwich, Conn, pp 93–120

Rattner JB, Rees J, Whitehead CM, Casiano CA, Tan EM, Humbel R-L, Conrad K, Fritzler MJ (1997) High frequency of neoplasia in patients with autoantibodies to centromere protein CENP-F. Clin Invest Med 20: 308–319

Reimer G, Raska I, Tan EM, Scheer U (1987) Human autoantibodies: probes for nucleolus structure and function. Virchows Arch B 54: 131–143

Rothfield NF (1992) Autoantibodies in scleroderma. Rheum Dis Clin North Am 18: 483–498

Rubin RL, Burlingame RW (1991) Biochemical mechanisms in autoimmunity. Biochem Soc Trans 19: 153–159

Saleem G, Li SC, MacPherson BR, Cooper SM (2001) Hepatitis with interference inflammation and IgG, IgM, and IgA anti-double-stranded DNA antibodies following inflixamab therapy: comment of article by Charles et al. Arthritis Rheum 44: 1966–1968

Selak S, Scheonroth L, Senécal J-L, Fritzler MJ (1999) Early endosome antigen 1: an autoantigen associated with neurological diseases. J Invest Med 47: 311–318

Slobbe RL, Pruijn GJM, Damen WGM, Van Der Kemp JWCM, Van Venrooij WJ (1991) Detection and occurrence of the 60-and 52-kD Ro-(SS-A) antigens and of autoantibodies against these proteins. Clin Exp Immunol 86: 99–105

Soussi T (2000) p53 antibodies in the sera of patients with various types of cancer: a review. Cancer Res 60: 1777–1788

Stokes DL, Griffin GD, Vo-Dinh T (2001) Detection of *E. coli* using a microfluidics-based antibody biochip detection system. Fresenius J Anal Chem 369: 295–301

Stollar BD (1990) The origin and pathogenic role of anti-DNA antibodies. Curr Opin Immunol 2: 607–612

Stone M, Salomen D, Lax B, Payne U, Lapp V, Inman R (2001) Clinical and imaging correlates of response to treatment with inflixamab in patients with ankylosing spondylitis. J Rheumatol 28: 1605–1614

Takano S, Matsushima H, Hiwatashi T, Miyachi K (1989) Detection of anti-SS-A/Ro antibody by using pig spleen supernatant and characterization of corresponding antigen. 2(1): 67–78

Takeuchi K, Turley SJ, Tan EM, Pollard KM (1995) Analysis of the autoantibody response to fibrillarin in human disease and murine models of autoimmunity. J Immunol 154: 961–971

Tan EM (1989) Antinuclear antibodies: diagnostic markers for autoimmune diseases and probes for cell biology. Adv Immunol 44: 93–151

Tan EM (1991) Autoantibodies in pathology and cell biology. Cell 67: 841–842

Tan EM (1999) Autoantibodies in diagnosis and identifying autoantigens. Immunologist 7: 85–92

Tan EM, Smolen JS, McDougal JS, Klippel JH, Fritzler MJ, Gordon TP, Hardin JA, Kalden JR, Lahita RG, Maini RN, Rothfield NF, Takasaki Y, Wiik A, Wilson MR, Koziol JA (2002) A critical evaluation of enzyme immunoassay kits for the detection of antinuclear antibodies of defined specificities II: potential for quantitation of antibody content. J Rheumatol 29: 68–74

Tseng CE, Buyon JP (1997) Neonatal lupus syndromes. Rheum Dis Clin North Am 23: 31–54

Tseng CE, Caldwell K, Feit S, Chan EKL, Buyon JP (1996) Subclass distribution of maternal and neonatal anti-Ro(SSA) and La(SSB) antibodies in congenital heart block. J Rheumatol 23: 925–932 van Bruggen MC, Kramers C, Hylkema MN, Smeenk RJ, Berden JH (1994) Pathophysiology of lupus nephritis: the role of nucleosomes. Neth J Med 45: 273–279

Verthelyi D, Ahmed SA (1999) Characterization of estrogen-induced autoantibodies to cardiolipin in non-autoimmune mice. Autoimmunity 10: 115–125

von Muhlen CA, Tan EM (1995) Autoantibodies in the diagnosis of systemic rheumatic disease. Semin Arthritis Rheum 24: 323–358

von Muhlen CA, Chan EKL, Anglés-Cano E, Mamula MJ, Garcia-de la Torre I, Fritzler MJ (1998) Advances in autoantibodies in SLE. Lupus 7: 507–514

Waite RL, Sentry JW, Stenmark H, Toh BH (1998) Autoantibodies to a novel early endosome antigen 1. Clin Immunol Immunopathol 86: 81–87

Wolin SL, Steitz JA (1984) The Ro small cytoplasmic ribonucleoproteins: identification of the antigenic protein and its binding site on the Ro RNAs. Proc Natl Acad Sci USA 81: 1996–2000

Woolley AT (2001) Biomedical microdevices and nanotechnology. Trends Biotechnol 19: 38–39

Xia P, Fritz KA, Geoghegan WD, Jordon RE (1987) The particulate (speckled-like thread) nuclear staining pattern: species and cellular distribution of the Ro/SS-A antigen. J Clin Lab Immunol 22: 101–105

Yang JM, Baserga SJ, Turley SJ, Pollard KM (2001) Fibrillarin and other snoRNP proteins are targets of autoantibodies in xenobiotic-induced autoimmunity. Clin Immunol 101: 38–50

Leflunomide therapy for autoimmune diseases

Angela Gause*, Claudia Metzler, Eva Reinhold-Keller, and Wolfgang L. Gross

Poliklinik für Rheumatologie, Universitätsklinikum Lübeck, Lübeck and Innere Medizin/Rheumatologie/Klinische Immunologie, Rheumaklinik Bad Bramstedt, Bad Bramstedt

Introduction

Leflunomide has been shown to be an effective drug for the treatment of inflammatory arthritis in animal models and in humans. By its action on the enzyme dehydro-orotat-dehydrogenase it interferes with pyrimidine nucleoside biosynthesis and acts on the proliferation of activated lymphocytes (Fox et al. 1999, Case 2001). Because of its immunomodulatory actions it is a drug which will be interesting also for other autoimmune diseases; further mechanisms beside the lymphocyte inhibitory effect may contribute to its effectiveness. The scope of this article is not a complete review of mechanisms and applications of leflunomide but a summary of new insights in action and applications in autoimmune diseases other than rheumatoid arthritis for further potential use.

Mechanisms of action

The most important mechanism of action of the active metabolite of leflunomide A77 1726 is its inhibition of proliferating lymphocytes. By inhibition of pyrimidine synthesis the cell cycle progression through the S phase is inhibited. The antiproliferative effect of leflunomide is working on T as well as on B lymphocytes, hereby inhibiting T-dependent as well as T-independent antibody production (Siemasko et al. 1996).

Recently it has been shown that the effect on immune cells is important also for the clinical downregulation of inflammation in patients with rheumatoid

* Author's address: Poliklinik für Rheumatologie, Universitätsklinikum Lübeck, Retzeburger Allee 160, 23538 Lübeck, Federal Republic of Germany.
E-mail: a.gause@ukl.mu-luebeck.de

arthritis. In the investigation by Kraan et al. (2000) patients receiving leflunomide for the treatment of active rheumatoid arthritis underwent synovial biopsies before and 4 weeks after the start of treatment with leflunomide. In 16 patients, synovial biopsies before and after 16 weeks of treatment with leflunomide were investigated for cellular infiltrates, adhesion molecules, cytokines, and matrix metalloproteinase 1 (MMP-1) and its inhibitor (TIMP-1): overall cellularity decreased significantly as well as macrophages in the sublining, intercellular and vascular cell adhesion molecule-1 (ICAM-1 and VCAM-1) expression, and MMP-1 and TIMP-1 expression. Of special interest was the comparative analysis of these markers in clinical responders and nonresponders to leflunomide treatment: the leflunomide responders displayed a reduction of ICAM-1, VCAM-1, and tumor necrosis factor alpha (TNF-α) expression, while the nonresponders had an increase in ICAM-1, TNF-α and interleukin-1β expression. Also the MMP-1-to-TIMP-1 ratio as a marker of destructive capacity of matrix-metalloproteinase was reduced more than 8-fold in the responders compared to the nonresponders of leflunomide therapy.

In vitro an effective downregulation of TNF-α-mediated inflammatory reactions has been shown. In transfected HeLa cells, nuclear factor κB-dependent reporter gene expression induced by TNF, TNFR1, TRAF2, and NIK was inhibited by A77 1726 in a dose-dependent manner that was also inhibitable by addition of uridine (Manna et al. 2000). This suppression of signal transduction was also shown in Jurkat cells, a human T-cell line and in human peripheral blood lymphocytes. Further it was shown that IκBα phosphorylation and IκBα kinase as well as activator protein-1 activation was inhibited by addition of A771726. These are all mechanisms which may explain the immunosuppressive action of leflunomide in vivo. In contrast, the induction of apoptosis, which is also induced by TNF-α, was significantly inhibited by leflunomide. Main inflammatory actions of TNF-α, the induction of lipid peroxidation and the production of reactive oxygen species, were also efficiently downregulated by the addition of the active metabolite A771726 to cell cultures. All these effects were, however, not mediated by TNFR1, because TNF-α and TNFR1 interaction was not inhibited.

Antiviral action of leflunomide

Experiences with leflunomide as an experimental drug for immunosuppression in transplantation led to the observation that the active metabolite has in vitro an antiviral effect on cytomegalovirus and herpes simplex virus type 1 production. Cytomegalovirus production by endothelial cells and fibroblasts in vitro was inhibited in a dose-dependent manner over a range of pharmacologically relevant concentrations of A771726. Apparently it does not act on the assembly of the virions by inhibition of viral synthesis like currently used antiviral drugs (Knight et al. 2001). These findings have been extended to experiments with herpes simplex virus. Furthermore, activity against cytomegalovirus could also be shown in a rat animal model (Waldman et al. 1999).

Clinical application other than rheumatoid arthritis

Leflunomide in Felty's syndrome

A single case of Felty's syndrome, a 56-year-old man with a 26-year history of rheumatoid arthritis, is published. Leflunomide was started when the patient had an absolute neutrophil count of $272/mm^3$ and a white blood cell count of $1700/mm^3$ (no large granular lymphocytes). Over the following 6 months, cell counts recovered to $1602/mm^3$ for neutrophils and $3000/mm^3$ for total white leukocytes, rheumatoid arthritis improved and prednisone could be discontinued (Talip et al. 2001).

Leflunomide in bullous pemphigoid

In two patients with bullous pemphigoid who were responsive only to high doses of prednisone and could not be tapered to a daily dose of prednisone below 20 mg, leflunomide was used in a dose of 20 mg daily successfully so that the prednisone could be discontinued. The patients remained in a clinical remission after a reduction of their respective leflunomide dose to 10 mg daily and 10 mg every other day (Nousari and Anhalt 2000).

Leflunomide in Wegener's granulomatosis

A larger experience exists with the use of leflunomide for the maintenance of remission in Wegener's granulomatosis (WG). This disease is firstly characterized by a granulomatous inflammation of the upper airways with a predominant Th1 immune reaction. In the generalized phase of the disease with dangerous life-threatening organ manifestations, a characteristic antibody against proteinase 3 (PR3) localized in the cytoplasm of neutrophils is found (Gross et al. 2000). In the generalized form of WG this antibody has a diagnostic specificity of more than 95% (Hagen et al. 1998, Choi et al. 2001), furthermore antineutrophil cytoplasmic antibodies (ANCA) have been shown to have a local proinflammatory activity in the blood vessels (Radford et al. 2000, Sibelius et al. 1998). Standard treatment for the acute phase is cyclophosphamide, which cannot be used for long-term treatment because of its long-term toxicity (Reinhold-Keller et al. 2000). Because of frequent relapses of WG, a "milder" immunosuppressive treatment for maintenance of remission as alternative to azathioprine and methotrexate is needed (de Groot et al. 1996, Langford and Sneller 2001).

In an open-label, single-center investigation 20 patients with generalized WG were treated with leflunomide after successful induction of remission with standard cyclophosphamide-prednisone combination therapy (Metzler et al. 1999). All patients started leflunomide with the 100 mg daily loading dose and following daily doses of 20 mg for 12 weeks. Concomitant low-dose prednisone was allowed during the study. Thereafter an efficacy assessment was performed followed by a dose escalation with a new loading dose of 100 mg of leflunomide for 2 days and an increase of the daily dose of leflunomide to 30 mg. After 24 weeks an efficacy assessment was performed again and those patients who had not yet

Table 1. Overview of the presently performed investigation of leflunomide versus methotrexate for maintenance of remission in WG

Aim
Comparison of leflunomide and methotrexate for maintenance of remission, prospectively, randomized, leflunomide (20–30 mg/day) vs. methotrexate (15–20 mg/week)

Inclusion criteria
120 WG patients in remission induced by cyclophosphamide (adapted from Fauci); max. steroid dose needed, 10 mg of prednisolone per day

Exclusion criteria
Serum creatinine above 1.3 mg/dl, usual contraindications against methotrexate and leflunomide

achieved complete remission were treated with daily 40 mg of leflunomide after another 100 mg dose for 2 days. In the 2.5 years of the study only one patient suffered a severe relapse with the necessity to reintroduce cyclophosphamide-prednisone. There were no minor relapses (increased WG activity), defined as the necessity to increase the leflunomide to improve treatment efficacy prior to the protocol-specified time points at 12 and 24 weeks. A total number of eight minor relapses defined as recurrent or new organ involvement occurred mostly after the first year of leflunomide treatment. One major relapse required treatment with cyclophosphamide-prednisone. The most frequently observed adverse events were upper airway infection (40%), followed by arthralgia and hypertension (35% each), dry skin, nail disorders, diarrhea, and vasculitis (30% each). Most adverse events were mild and moderate, only 2 patients experienced serious adverse events, one a severe pneumonia and the other a visual field defect. In summary, the overall efficacy was judged so good that a controlled randomized investigation comparing leflunomide to low-dose weekly methotrexate has been started now as a project of the German Competence Network Rheumatology (Kompetenznetz Rheuma) (Table 1).

Further perspectives

In the light of the recent success with the introduction of TNF-α blocking agents into the treatment of WG (Gause 2001, Stone et al. 2001), leflunomide might be of special value for maintenance of remission by its potential to block TNF after achieving a remission with a combination of cyclophosphamide and a biological TNF blocker. A clinical example is the following case.

A 59-year-old man presented with a PR3-ANCA-positive pulmonary renal syndrome as first WG manifestation accompanied by an occlusion of the left central ocular artery because of temporal giant cell arteritis. After remission-inducing therapy with cyclophosphamide and prednisone for 11 months and a methotrexate maintenance therapy for 11 months he suffered a renal relapse with progressive glomerulonephritis (rise of serum creatinine from 1.3 to 3.1 mg/dl, dysmorphic hematuria) which was refractory to the standard treatment with cyclophosphamide and prednisone. After four infusions of infliximab (3 mg/kg of weight over 14 weeks;

Table 2. Successful induction of remission in a severe case of generalized WG refractory to standard therapy with the TNF-α-blocking chimeric antibody infliximab and subsequent maintenance of remission with leflunomide. During leflunomide treatment kidney function recovered further and prednisolone therapy could be tapered down and stopped

Time	11/99	12/99	01/00	02/00	03/00	04/00	06/00	10/00	02/01	08/01	11/01
Infliximab (3 mg/kg)		Inf	Inf	Inf	Inf						
Leflunomide (mg/d)						20	30	30	30	30	30
Prednisolone (mg/d)	250	50	30	20	15	10	10	6.25	5	2	0
Cyclophosphamide (mg/d)	200	100	100	75	75	75					
Active sediment	+	++	++	−	−	−	−	−	−	−	−
Creatinine (mg/dl)	1.7	3.1	2.8	3.2	2.2	2.1	2.1	1.9	1.8	1.7	1.6
cANCA (titer)	1:512	1:512	1:128	1:128	1:64	neg.	neg.	neg.	neg.	neg.	neg.

week 0, 2, 6, and 12) a remission was achieved (serum creatinine, 2.0 mg/dl; glomerular filtration rate, 42 ml/min). For maintenance of remission, leflunomide was started in a daily dose of 20 mg and increased to 30 mg/day after two months. In the following 20 months no further relapse occurred and the patient's serum creatinine recovered further to 1.6 mg/dl. Daily prednisolone was discontinued. Serum ANCA titer turned to negative during the TNF-α blocking therapy and stayed negative under leflunomide (Table 2). We speculate that the TNF-blocking capacity of leflunomide might be active also in vivo and that it therefore might be especially efficient in those WG cases responsive to biological TNF-α antagonists.

In summary, besides its proven efficacy in rheumatoid arthritis, leflunomide has immunomodulatory and probably antiviral capacities that can be used for the long-term treatment of autoimmune diseases. Further investigations have been started in WG and may be feasible also for other types of systemic vasculitis, e.g., Churg–Strauss syndrome and temporal arteritis or other diseases like pemphigus vulgaris.

References

Case JP (2001) Old and new drugs used in rheumatoid arthritis: a historical perspective. Part 2: the newer drugs and drug strategies. Am J Ther 8: 163–179

Choi HK, Liu S, Merkel PA, Colditz GA, Niles JL (2001) Diagnostic performance of antineutrophil cytoplasmic antibody tests for idiopathic vasculitides: metaanalysis with a focus on antimyeloperoxidase antibodies. J Rheumatol 28: 1584–1590

de Groot K, Reinhold-Keller E, Tatsis E, Paulsen J, Heller M, Nölle B, Gross WL (1996) Therapy for the maintenance of remission in sixty-five patients with generalized Wegener's granulomatosis: methotrexate versus trimethoprim/sulfamethoxazole. Arthritis Rheum 39: 2052–2061

Fox RI, Herrmann ML, Frangou CG, Wahl GM, Morris RE, Kirschbaum BJ (1999) How does leflunomide modulate the immune response in rheumatoid arthritis? BioDrugs 12: 301–315

Gause AL, Lamprecht P, Voswinkel J, Lilienthal T, Gross WL (2001) Effectiveness of TNF-alpha blockade with infliximab in refractory Wgener's granulomatosis. Clin Immunol 99: 176

Gross WL, Trabandt A, Reinhold-Keller E (2000) Diagnosis and evaluation of vasculitis. Rheumatology 39: 245–252

Hagen EC, Daha MR, Hermans J, Andrassy K, Csernok E, Gaskin G, Lesavre P, Lüdemann J, Rasmussen N, Sinico RA, Wiik A, van der Woude FJ (1998) Diagnostic value of standardized assays for anti-neutrophil cytoplasmic antibodies in idiopathic systemic vasculitis: EC/BCR project for ANCA assay standardization. Kidney Int 53: 743–753

Knight DA, Hejmanowski AQ, Dierksheide JE, Williams JW, Chong AS, Waldman WJ (2001) Inhibition of herpes simplex virus type 1 by the experimental immunosuppressive agent leflunomide. Transplantation 71: 170–174

Kraan MC, Reece RJ, Barg EC, Smeets TJM, Farnell J, Rosenburg R, Veale DJ, Breedveld FC, Emery P, Tak PP (2000) Modulation of inflammation and metalloproteinase expression in synovial tissue by leflunomide and methotrexate in patients with active rheumatoid arthritis: findings in a prospective, randomized, double-blind, parallel-design clinical trial in thirty-nine patients at two centers. Arthritis Rheum 43: 1820–1830

Langford CA, Sneller MC (2001) Update on the diagnosis and treatment of Wegener's granulomatosis. Adv Intern Med 46: 177–206

Manna SK, Mukhopadhyay A, Aggarwal BB (2000) Leflunomide suppresses TNF-induced cellular responses: effects on NF-kappa B, activator protein-1, c-Jun N-terminal protein kinase, and apoptosis. J Immunol 165: 5962–5969

Metzler C, Loew-Friedrich J, Reinhold-Keller E, Fink C, Lamprecht P, Gross WL (1999) Maintenance of remission with leflunomide in Wegener's granulomatosis. Arthritis Rheum 42 Suppl: 1466

Nousari HC, Anhalt GJ (2000) Bullous pemphigoid treated with leflunomide: a novel immunomodulatory agent. Arch Dermatol 136: 1204–1205

Radford DJ, Savage CO, Nash GB (2000) Treatment of rolling neutrophils with antineutrophil cytoplasmic antibodies causes conversion to firm integrin-mediated adhesion. Arthritis Rheum 43: 1337–1345

Reinhold-Keller E, Beuge N, Latza U, de Groot K, Rudert K, Nölle B, Heller M, Gross WL (2000) An interdisciplinary approach to the care of patients with Wegener's granulomatosis: long-term outcome in 155 patients. Arthritis Rheum 43: 1021–1032

Sibelius U, Hattar K, Schenkel A, Noll T, Csernok E, Gross WL, Mayet WJ, Piper HM, Seeger W, Grimminger F (1998) Wegener's granulomatosis: anti-proteinase 3 antibodies are potent inductors of human endothelial cell signaling and leakage response. J Exp Med 187: 497–503

Siemasko KF, Chong AS, Williams JW, Bremer EG, Finnegan A (1996) Regulation of B cell function by the immunosuppressive agent leflunomide. Transplantation 61: 635–642

Stone JH, Uhlfelder ML, Hellmann DB, Crook S, Bedocs NM, Hoffman GS (2001) Etanercept combined with conventional treatment in Wegener's granulomatosis: a six-month open-label trial to evaluate safety. Arthritis Rheum 44: 1149–1154

Talip F, Walker N, Khan W, Zimmermann B (2001) Treatment of Felty's syndrome with leflunomide. J Rheumatol 28: 868–870

Waldman WJ, Knight DA, Blinder L, Shen J, Lurain NS, Miller DM, Sedmak DD, Williams JW, Chong AS (1999) Inhibition of cytomegalovirus in vitro and in vivo by the experimental immunosuppressive agent leflunomide. Intervirology 42: 412–418

Immunotherapy for ocular inflammatory disease

Kathrin H. Greiner and **John V. Forrester***

Department of Ophthalmology, Medical School, Aberdeen Royal Infirmary,
Aberdeen, United Kingdom

Experimental uveitis models

Uveitis has been defined as inflammation of the uveal tract (iris, ciliary body, or choroid). More recently it has been recharacterised as intraocular inflammation (IOI) since many forms of uveitis involve intraocular structures such as the retina, vitreous, and even the lens (Forrester et al. 1998).

Inflammation may be restricted to the eye or the eye may be involved in many ways as part of a systemic disease (e.g., multisystem connective tissue). Usually one or more of the ocular coats are affected by an inflammatory process. IOI in arthritic disease may be linked to infectious diseases, as seen in the triad of Yersinia enterocolitis, ankylosing spondylitis (AS), and uveitis. Indeed, the possible association between such disease clusters and pathogenetic mechanisms involving infectious agents, autoimmunity, and molecular mimicry is actively under investigation, particularly with regard to the role of major histocompatibility (MHC) class I antigens in susceptibility to disease.

Classification of intraocular inflammation (uveitis) according to anatomic location differentiates between anterior-segment intraocular inflammation (ASII, anterior uveitis), posterior-segment intraocular inflammation (PSII, posterior uveitis), and combined anterior- and posterior-segment intraocular inflammation (panuveitis). Pathogenetically, ASII is recognised to be more closely associated with MHC class I antigens such as HLA B27, which rely on CD8$^+$ T cells, and a foreign or autoantigen, although the nature of such antigens remains to be determined. PSII in contrast is much less clearly associated with MHC class I antigens. In contrast, PSII as studied experimentally requires MHC class II (on antigen-presenting cells [APCs]) CD4$^+$ T cells and putative autoantigens located in the retina or lens but which clinically are still unknown (Fig. 1).

* Authors' address: Department of Ophthalmology, Medical School, Aberdeen Royal Infirmary, Foresterhill, Aberdeen AB25 2ZA, United Kingdom.

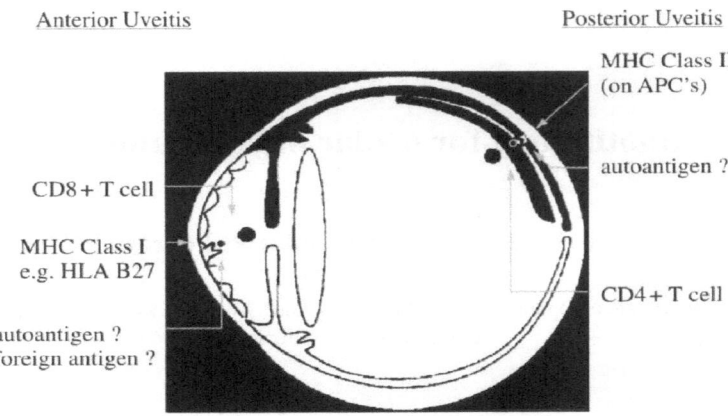

Fig. 1. Pathogenetic classification of uveitis

There can be variable "spillover" into the anterior segment (Forrester 1990) with posterior-segment disease. ASII is most frequently an acute, recurrent illness involving the iris and ciliary body and may occur as an HLA-B27$^+$ or an HLA-B27$^-$ disease (Feltkamp et al. 1994). Chronic forms of ASII also occur, as with systemic disease (e.g., juvenile seronegative arthritis), but are much less common. PSII, by contrast, has a high degree of heterogeneity and presents with a variety of clinical syndromes of markedly different severity and visual consequences. Despite this, it is now increasingly recognized that many forms of PSII are part of a spectrum of uveoretinal inflammatory disease (Forrester et al. 1990).

The four typical signs of PSII are vitreous cells, vasculitis, edema, and chorioretinal microgranulomata (Fig. 2). In many cases the etiology of PSII is not clear. These cases are often presumed to be noninfectious, endogenous forms of inflammation. This group includes eye inflammations associated with systemic disease

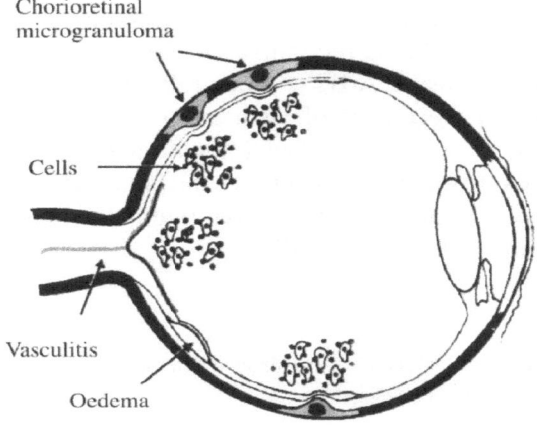

Fig. 2. The four signs of posterior uveitis

Table 1. Experimental models of autoimmune uveitis

Experimental model	Antigen	Epitopes (n)
Autoimmune uveoretinitis (EAU)	S antigen	>4 (M, N, K, L, 680)
	IRBP	>4
	rhodopsin	1
	recoverin	?
	phosducin	?
Melanin-induced uveitis (EMIU)	melanin-associated proteins (e.g., TRP1, TRP2)	
Autoimmune uveitis	PEP-65	
Anterior chamber assn uveitis (EAAU)	RPE protein	

such as systemic lupus erythematosus or sarcoidosis. In some cases such as toxoplasma retinochorioiditis, the etiology of PSII is clear and well documented.

Much of our understanding of the pathology of PSII has come from experimental models of uveoretinitis. Interestingly, in animal models a single antigen (such as retinal S-antigen or inter photoreceptor retinoid binding protein [IRBP]) can reproduce the full range of human presentations of PSII (Forrester et al. 1990). Merely by modifying the species or strain of animal, the immunological status of the animal or dose of the antigen, the full spectrum of clinicopathological conditions can be induced (Forrester 1990, 1991, 1992). For instance, S-antigen will produce signs of retinal vasculitis in the monkey and exudative retinal detachment in the Lewis rat (Forrester et al. 1990). The same antigen can induce a syndrome of low-grade focal "white-dot" infiltrates with subretinal neovascularization resembling various forms of PSII in the B10A mouse (Caspi et al. 1992). It appears therefore that the posterior segment of the eye responds to autoimmune or infectious insults in similar ways, the clinical appearance depending on the genetic makeup of the individual (Caspi et al. 1992) and the immunological status as much as upon the nature and dose of the foreign or self antigen. Even though each inflammatory eye condition may have its own characteristic presentation, these concepts help us to understand the high degree of overlap between clinical syndromes and why one condition can progress to another clinical entity over time.

An overview of the commonly used uveitis animal models is given in Table 1. Experimental autoimmune uveoretinitis (EAU) induced by IRBP represents a disease similar to clinical chorioretinitis and has served for many years as the central model for human ocular inflammation of presumed autoimmune origin.

Mucosal tolerance

Administration of antigens, including autoantigens, via the mucosal tract (gut, respiratory, or conjunctival) results in the development of a state of peripheral immunological tolerance (Xiao and Link 1997). At the same dose, mucosal tolerance is more effective after nasal compared to oral administration of antigens (Shi et al. 1999). The effect of nasal tolerance with IRBP has been investigated in the EAU mouse model. It has been shown that the amount of inflammatory cells and structural tissue damage were markedly reduced in animals tolerized by either a single dose of 10 or 30 µg of IRBP as compared to control animals treated with phosphate-buffered saline only (Jiang et al. 2001). Another experiment on nasal tolerance demonstrated that a single- or double-dose protocol can reduce EAU significantly, whereas a triple dose does not appear to limit the EAU activity (Jiang et al. 2001). This state of tolerance appears to rely on the induction of regulatory T cells since it can be adoptively transferred in Lewis rats with tolerized splenocytes to suppress retinal antigen-induced EAU. The effect of mucosal tolerance combined with immunosuppressive therapy such as cyclosporin A (CSA) or mycophenolate mofetil (MMF) has also been investigated. Interestingly, mucosal tolerization with retinal extract plus administration of CSA significantly delayed the expected day of EAU onset as compared with CSA alone or tolerization only (Kreutzer et al. 1997). However, there was no such combined effect of retinal extract applied via the nasal mucosa with the concurrent application of MMF (Dick et al. 1998). This has important clinical implications for the use of such therapies since many patients potentially eligible for tolerance induction protocols are usually also on treatment with immunosuppressants.

At least two mechanisms are operative in the mediation of oral tolerance: active suppression and clonal anergy/deletion. A number of factors such as antigen dose, antigen form, and the timing of antigen administration determine which mechanism of tolerance is operative. Work from these animal models has recently been extended into human clinical trials of uveitis with limited success (Nussenblatt et al. 1997). However, mucosal tolerance induction is related to the route of antigen administration (oral, nasal, parenteral). To broaden the effectiveness of mucosal tolerance, a combination of tolerogens with cytokines/cholera toxin B subunit might enhance suppression of clinical disease. However, there is a risk of worsening an ongoing autoimmune disease by mucosal antigen administration, which has been incompletely addressed. Many more studies are needed to define an effective and safe procedure to be used in humans.

Macrophage depletion

Macrophages appear to have a critical role from the onset of inflammation and are major effector cells in tissue damage. For instance, it has been shown that the effect of a tumor necrosis factor receptor (TNFr) fusion protein on reducing EAU severity in rats had a significant role in reducing macrophage infiltration into the issues compared to T cells (Dick et al. 1996). Therefore in separate experiments the role of macrophages was directly addressed. The effect of macrophage-specific blockade on EAU has been investigated using di-chloromethylene diphosphonate (Cl2MDP) (Forrester et al. 1998). It was shown that the clinical and histological uveitis scores were significantly lower in Cl2MDP-treated animals (Lewis rats) as compared to controls. Mannosylated liposomes had an even stronger effect than non-mannosylated liposomes on the suppression of uveitis. This can be explained by the fact that macrophages have mannose receptors and therefore took the drug up more readily (Forrester et al. 1998).

Antigen-presenting cells in the retina

Retinal pigment epithelial cells (Forrester et al. 1990), Müller/glial cells, endothelial cells (Wang et al. 1995), neurones, microglia (Zhang et al. 1997, Yang et al. 2000, Matsubara et al. 1999), and perivascular macrophages (Provis et al. 1996) have all been suggested as candidate APCs in the retina. However, at present only perivascular macrophages are still thought to represent APCs in the retina (on the basis of little direct evidence), whereas the before-mentioned cell types seem to be inhibitors to the immune response (Broderick et al. 2000). Antigen-presenting dendritic cells are found in the choroid but not the retina. Close approximation of these two layers may allow transfer of antigen from the photoreceptor–retinal pigment epithelial cell interface to the juxtaposed dendritic cells in the choroid and permit antigen transport to the site of the draining lymph nodes, where systemic activation of T cells can be induced. In addition, cross-reactivity with systemic foreign antigen may occur in the same draining lymph nodes thus promoting the induction of inflammation when the activated T cells traffick back to the site of injury in the tissues, i.e., the retina or uveal tract. Much more work is needed to dissect these processes, but already therapy of human uveitis or PSII has been developed on the basis of the results from these experimental models.

Treatment of human PSII

Overall therapeutic objectives

The aims of treatment are twofold. At the initial stages of the disease the immediate threat to sight needs to be removed. Corticosteroids act fastest and are therefore still the mainstay for the initial therapy of sight-threatening uveitis. However, they can cause a wide range of potentially serious side effects and are not suitable for long-term treatment at high doses. Immunosuppressives such as CSA or azathioprine have thus been introduced to provide long-term control of PSII, whereas topical treatment (corticosteroids, which reduce the inflammatory response, and mydriatics, which prevent the sequelae of the disease such as synechiae) is often sufficient in ASII. Adequate treatment is important since the inflammation can escape control and can cause, for instance, hypopyon uveitis and secondary glaucoma. Very rarely, systemic corticosteroids and systemic immunosuppression as for PSII may be necessary to treat severe acute anterior uveitis. This is particularly the case in juvenile idiopathic arthritis.

In the long term, the aim is to reduce immunosuppressive therapy to the minimal effective dose. This may be no therapy, CSA, or azathioprine alone or in combination with low dose steroids.

Immunosuppressants

CSA is an effective second-line treatment in noninfectious intraocular inflammation as well as a steroid sparing drug (Jabs et al. 2000). Its principal action is to suppress lymphokine production by T helper (Th) cells by interfering with the activation of lymphokine genes and, directly or indirectly, to reduce the expression of the receptors for interleukin-2 (IL-2r) on lymphocytes undergoing activation. CSA has recently been found to exert its therapeutic as well as side effects via the increased expression of transforming growth factor β (Khanna et al. 1999). Other macrolides such as tacrolimus and rapamycin also have immunosuppressive properties. Tacrolimus suppresses lymphokine production by Th cells in a manner similar to CSA, whereas rapamycin interferes with the intracellular signalling pathways of IL-2r and therefore prevents IL-2-dependent lymphocyte activation. Tacrolimus appears to have the advantage of a lower induction of arterial hypertension as compared with CSA, in which this is a common side effect. In a prospective, randomised, open-label, multicenter study on cardiac transplant patients, tacrolimus-based immunosuppression was shown to be associated with less hypertension and hyperlipidaemia and no difference in renal function, hyperglycaemia, or infection incidence when compared to cyclosporine-based immunosuppression (Taylor et al. 1999).

Other immunosuppressants, such as azathioprine, cyclophosphamide and chlorambucil, are within the spectrum of therapy, but each has significant side effects restricting its use. Additionally, some value has been obtained from the use of low-dose methotrexate, which is usually given as a once-weekly dose. The advantage of methotrexate is the extensive experience with and the relative safety of its use in children with juvenile rheumatoid arthritis (Wallace 1998). Methotrexate has also been used in patients with various ocular inflammatory diseases, including vasculitis, panuveitis, intermediate uveitis, vitritis, scleritis, orbital pseudotumor, myositis, and sarcoid-associated panuveitis (Holz et al. 1992, Shah et al. 1992, Dev et al. 1999).

Alternative therapies

In about one third of patients the inflammation will not be sufficiently controlled even with a combination of the above immunosuppressives. Over the last few years alternative therapies have therefore been developed with the aim to achieve more specificity and less side effects. One such immunosuppressive agent is MMF, which has been used to prevent allograft rejection in renal and cardiac transplantation but also as an effective agent in the treatment of ocular inflammatory diseases (Larkin and Lightman 1999, Kilmartin et al. 1998). MMF is commonly used in combination with other immunomodulatory drugs and appears to be an acceptable alternative to azathioprine or methotrexate, especially in patients intolerant of other agents. Reduction in uveitis activity during MMF therapy correlates with reduction in the frequency of peripheral blood CD69-positive CD4 cells (Kilmartin et al. 2001). The frequency of CD69-positive CD4 T cells is a measure of activity in posterior uveitis and may guide adequate immunosuppression (Kilmartin et al. 2001). One major advantage of MMF is its lack of nephrotoxicity and generally acceptable side effect profile.

Monoclonal-antibody therapies

However, the above therapies are relatively nonspecific. For this reason alternative therapies such as monoclonal-antibody therapy (e.g., anti-CD4, anti-Tac, anti-CD52) have been investigated (Smith et al. 1999) and are already used in selected cases in humans (Nussenblatt et al. 1999, Dick et al. 2000). Anti-IL-2 receptor antibody therapy, given in lieu of standard immunosuppressive therapy appeared to prevent the expression of severe sight-threatening intraocular inflammatory disease in 8 of 10 patients treated over a one-year period, with noted improvements in visual acuity (Nussenblatt et al. 1999). Another monoclonal antibody, Campath-1H, which recognises the pan-lymphocyte antigen CD52, is now licenced for use in chronic lymphatic leukaemia and has been used in patients with aggressive autoimmune and inflammatory diseases. In cases of severe refractory systemic vasculitis (Wegener's), remissions of several years were achieved (Lockwood et al. 1996). Single case studies have reported the success of Campath-1H therapy in controlling severe posterior uveitis (Isaacs et al. 1995) and in preventing recurrent corneal graft rejection (Newman et al. 1995) which were refractory to conventional immunosuppression. A further study on a cohort of ten patients with severe, refractory, noninfectious, immune-mediated, intraocular and orbital inflammatory disease treated with Campath-1H on a compassionate "named-patient" basis, underlines the effectiveness of its use (Dick et al. 2000). The disadvantage of Campath-1H is a lymphocytotoxic effect. While total peripheral blood lymphocyte numbers return to normal after therapy, there is a protracted reduction in $CD4^+$ peripheral blood lymphocyte counts, with inversion of the CD4-to-CD8 ratio.

Anti-TNF therapies

Another, currently still experimental treatment are anti-tumor necrosis factor (anti-TNF) therapies. These have been used extensively in rheumatoid arthritis, where they proved to be of great benefit (Moreland et al. 1997). Anti-TNF therapies can be in the form of anti-TNF antibodies or TNF fusion proteins (TNFr-Ig). Anti-TNF monoclonal antibody (infliximab) has successfully been used as a single infusion in five patients with sight-threatening panuveitis in Behcet's disease (Sfikakis et al. 2001). The authors reported remission of ocular inflammation within the first 24 h, and complete suppression 7 days after treatment in all patients without side effects (Sfikakis et al. 2001). TNF is a proinflammatory cytokine involved in the pathogenesis of inflammatory disease, and antagonism of TNF may reduce the activity of the disease. Production of TNF-α is associated with the synthesis and secretion of specific receptors, TNF-RI (55 kDa) and TNF-RII (75 kDa) (Tartaglia and Goeddel 1992). Both receptors are expressed on nearly all nucleated cell types and are thought to protect cells from TNF-α and to block the activity of this cytokine once it is released into the circulation (Van Zee et al. 1992, Hunger et al. 1997). Etanercept is a recombinant human TNF-α receptor-Fc fusion protein consisting of a dimer of the extracellular portion of two p75 TNF-α receptors fused to the Fc portion of human immunoglobulin G1. It has been used as a subcutaneous injection in 10 children with treatment-resistant uveitis who had failed previous therapy with topical steroids and methotrexate and/or cyclosporine. Within 3 months, 63% of affected eyes showed a rapid decrease in anterior chamber cell density, including remission of uveitis in 4 eyes. However, one child had an exacerbation of uveitis during Etanercept therapy (Reiff et al. 2001). Anti-TNF therapies can render patients less resistant to viral infections or other pathogens. Careful monitoring and prompt attention to any symptoms is important. Further potential problems with repeated use are the formation of anti-nuclear antibodies, rarely systemic lupus erythematosus-like reactions, and occasional lymphomas. Whereas the treatment results in patients with rheumatoid arthritis (Moreland et al. 1997) are very encouraging, further clinical trials to evaluate its potential in the treatment of uveitis patients are necessary and currently underway. At present, type and dose and frequency of TNFr-Ig application remain to be optimised and more patients will have to be treated before a reliable assessment of the effectiveness of these treatments in uveitis patients can be made. It is encouraging though that generally TNF inhibitors appear to be well-tolerated immunosuppressive medications that may benefit certain subgroups of patients with inflammatory eye disease (Smith et al. 2001, Reiff et al. 2001).

Future perspectives

Future developments are also aimed at developing new drug delivery systems, e.g., intravitreal steroid or cyclosporine implants (Jaffe et al. 1998) and iontophoresis-aided steroid delivery to the eye, that may avoid systemic side effects while providing long-term therapeutic effect of up to several years. Tolerance induction via mucosal immunisation (Dick et al. 1994, Nussenblatt et al. 1997) has also been evaluated but is mostly in the experimental realm at present due to the above-mentioned problems. The development of new biologicals (e.g., new anticytokines) which are more specific and better tolerated may be a promising alternative in the future. On the other hand, new methods to monitor patients, e.g., to recognise flare-ups earlier (CD69) and treat accordingly are needed.

References

Broderick C, Duncan L, Taylor N, Dick AD (2000) IFN-gamma and LPS-mediated IL-10-dependent suppression of retinal microglial activation. Invest Ophthalmol Vis Sci 41: 2613–2622

Caspi RR, Grubbs BG, Chan CC, Chader GJ, Wiggert B (1992) Genetic control of susceptibility to experimental autoimmune uveoretinitis in the mouse model. J Immunol 148: 2384–2389

Dev S, McCallum RM, Jaffe GJ (1999) Methotrexate treatment for sarcoid-associated panuveitis. Ophthalmology 106: 111–118

Dick AD, Cheng YF, Liversidge J, Forrester JV (1994) Intranasal administration of retinal antigens suppresses retinal antigen-induced experimental autoimmune uveoretinitis. Immunology 82: 625–631

Dick AD, McMenamin PG, Korner H, Scallon BJ, Ghrayeb J, Forrester JV, Sedgwick JD (1996) Inhibition of tumor necrosis factor activity minimizes target organ damage in experimental autoimmune uveoretinitis despite quantitatively normal activated T cell traffic to the retina. Eur J Immunol 26: 1018–1025

Dick AD, Kreutzer B, Laliotou B, Forrester JV (1998) Effects of mycophenolate mofetil on nasal mucosal tolerance induction. Invest Ophthalmol Vis Sci 39: 835–840

Dick AD, Meyer P, James T, Forrester JV, Hale G, Waldmann H, Isaacs JD (2000) Campath-1H therapy in refractory ocular inflammatory disease. Br J Ophthalmol 84: 107–109

Feltkamp TEW, BreurVriesendorp BS, Derhaag PJFM (1994) HLA-B27 subtypes and acute anterior uveitis: a review. Reg Immunol 6: 8–11

Forrester JV (1990) Uveitis. Br J Ophthalmol 74: 620–622

Forrester JV (1991) Uveitis: pathogenesis. Lancet 338(8781): 1498–1501

Forrester JV (1992) Duke-Elder Lecture: new concepts on the role of autoimmunity in the pathogenesis of uveitis. Eye 6 (Pt 5): 433–446

Forrester JV, Liversidge J, Dua HS (1990a) Regulation of the local immune response by retinal cells. Curr Eye Res 9 Suppl: 183–191

Forrester JV, Liversidge JM, Dua HS, Towler HM, McMenamin PG (1990b) Comparison of clinical and experimental uveitis. Curr Eye Res 9 Suppl: 75–84

Forrester JV, Okada AA, BenEzra D, Ohno S (1998a). In: Forrester JV, Okada AA, BenEzra D, Ohno S (eds) Posterior segment intraocular inflammation: guidelines. Kugler Publications, The Hague, The Netherlands, pp 3–7

Forrester JV, Huitinga I, Lumsden L, Dijkstra CD (1998b) Marrow-derived activated macrophages are required during the effector phase of experimental autoimmune uveoretinitis in rats. Curr Eye Res 17: 426–437

Holz FG, Krastel H, Breitbart A, Schwarz-Eywill M, Pezzutto A, Volcker HE (1992) Low-dose methotrexate treatment in non-infectious uveitis resistant to corticosteroids. Ger J Ophthalmol 1: 142–144

Hunger RE, Carnaud C, Garcia I, Vassalli P, Mueller C (1997) Prevention of autoimmune diabetes mellitus in NOD mice by transgenic expression of soluble tumor necrosis factor receptor p55. Eur J Immunol 27: 255–261

Isaacs JD, Hale G, Waldmann H, Dick AD, Haynes R, Forrester JV, Watson P, Meyer PA (1995) Monoclonal antibody therapy of chronic intraocular inflammation using campath-1H. Br J Ophthalmol 79: 1054–1055

Jabs DA, Rosenbaum JT, Foster CS, Holland GN, Jaffe GJ, Louie JS, Nussenblatt RB, Stiehm ER, Tessler H, Van Gelder RN, Whitcup SM, Yocum D (2000) Guidelines for the use of immunosuppressive drugs in patients with ocular inflammatory disorders: recommendations of an expert panel. Am J Ophthalmol 130: 492–513

Jaffe GJ, Yang CS, Want XC, Cousins SW, Gallemore RP, Ashton P (1998) Intravitreal sustained-release cyclosporin in the treatment of experimental uveitis. Ophthalmology 105: 46

Jiang HR, Taylor N, Duncan L, Dick AD, Forrester JV (2001) Total dose and frequency of administration critically affect success of nasal mucosal tolerance induction. Br J Ophthalmol 85: 739–744

Khanna AK, Cairns VR, Becker CG, Hosenpud JD (1999) Transforming growth factor (TGF)-beta mimics and anti-TGF-beta antibody abrogates the in vivo effects of cyclosporine: demonstration of a direct role of TGF-beta in immunosuppression and nephrotoxicity of cyclosporine. Transplantation 67: 882–889

Kilmartin DJ, Forrester JV, Dick AD (1998) Rescue therapy with mycophenolate mofetil in refractory uveitis. Lancet 352: 35–36

Kilmartin DJ, Fletcher ZJ, Almeida JA, Liversidge J, Forrester JV, Dick AD (2001) CD69 expression on peripheral CD4$^+$ T cells parallels disease activity and is reduced by mycophenolate mofetil therapy in uveitis. Invest Ophthalmol Vis Sci 42: 1285–1292

Kreutzer B, Laliotou B, Cheng YF, Liversidge J, Forrester JV, Dick AD (1997) Nasal administration of retinal antigens maintains immunosuppression of uveoretinitis in cyclosporin-A-treated Lewis rats: future treatment of endogenous posterior uveoretinitis? Eye 11 (Pt 4): 445–452

Larkin G, Lightman S (1999) Mycophenolate mofetil: a useful immunosuppressive in inflammatory eye disease. Ophthalmology 106: 370–374

Lockwood CM, Thiru S, Stewart S, Hale G, Isaacs J, Wraight P, Elliott J, Waldmann H (1996) Treatment of refractory Wegeners granulomatosis with humanised monoclonal antibodies. Q J Med 89: 903–912

Matsubara T, Pararajasegaram G, Wu GS, Rao NA (1999) Retinal microglia differentially express phenotypic markers of antigen-presenting cells in vitro. Invest Ophthalmol Vis Sci 40: 3186–3193

Moreland LW, Baumgartner SW, Schiff MH, Tindall EA, Fleischmann RM, Weaver AL, Ettlinger RE, Cohen S, Koopman WJ, Mohler K, Widmer MB, Blosch CM (1997) Treatment of rheumatoid arthritis with a recombinant human tumor necrosis factor receptor (p75)-Fc fusion protein. N Engl J Med 337: 141–147

Newman DK, Isaacs JD, Watson PG, Meyer PA, Hale G, Waldmann H (1995) Prevention of immune-mediated corneal graft destruction with the anti-lymphocyte monoclonal antibody, Campath-1H. Eye 9: 564–569

Nussenblatt RB, Whitcup SM, de Smet MD, Caspi RR, Kozhich AT, Weiner HL, Vistica B, Gery I (1996) Intraocular inflammatory disease (uveitis) and the use of oral tolerance: a status report. Ann N Y Acad Sci 778: 325–337

Nussenblatt RB, Gery I, Weiner HL, Ferris FL, Shiloach J, Remaley N, Perry C, Caspi RR, Hafler DA, Foster CS, Whitcup SM (1997) Treatment of uveitis by oral administration of retinal antigens: results of a phase I/II randomized masked trial. Am J Ophthalmol 123: 583–592

Nussenblatt RB, Fortin E, Schiffman R, Rizzo L, Smith J, Van Veldhuisen P, Sran P, Yaffe A, Goldman CK, Waldmann TA, Whitcup SM (1999) Treatment of noninfectious intermediate and posterior uveitis with the humanized anti-Tac mAb: a phase I/II clinical trial. Proc Natl Acad Sci USA 96: 7462–7466

Provis JM, Diaz CM, Penfold PL (1996) Microglia in human retina: a heterogeneous population with distinct ontogenies. Perspect Dev Neurobiol 3: 213–222

Reiff A, Takei S, Sadeghi S, Stout A, Shaham B, Bernstein B, Gallagher K, Stout T (2001) Etanercept therapy in children with treatment-resistant uveitis. Arthritis Rheum 44: 1411–1415

Sfikakis PP, Theodossiadis PG, Katsiari CG, Kaklamanis P, Markomichelakis NN (2001) Effect of infliximab on sight-threatening panuveitis in Behcet's disease. Lancet 358(9278): 295–296

Shah SS, Lowder CY, Schmitt MA, Wilke WS, Kosmorsky GS, Meisler DM (1992) Low-dose methotrexate therapy for ocular inflammatory disease. Ophthalmology 99: 1419–1423

Shi FD, Li H, Wang H, Bai X, van der Meide PH, Link H, Ljunggren HG (1999) Mechanisms of nasal tolerance induction in experimental autoimmune myasthenia gravis: identification of regulatory cells. J Immunol 162: 5757–5763

Smith JR, Hart PH, Parish CR, Standfield SD, Coster DJ, Williams KA (1999) Experimental melanin-induced uveitis in the Fischer 344 rat is inhibited by anti-CD4 monoclonal antibody, but not by mannose-6-phosphate. Clin Exp Immunol 115: 64–71

Smith JR, Levinson RD, Holland GN, Jabs DA, Robinson MR, Whitcup SM, Rosenbaum JT (2001) Differential efficacy of tumor necrosis factor inhibition in the management of inflammatory eye disease and associated rheumatic disease. Arthritis Rheum 45: 252–257

Tartaglia LA, Goeddel DV (1992) Two TNF receptors. Immunol Today 13: 151–153

Taylor DO, Barr ML, Radovancevic B, Renlund DG, Mentzer RM Jr, Smart FW, Tolman DE, Frazier OH, Young JB, VanVeldhuisen P (1999) A randomized, multicenter comparison of tacrolimus and cyclosporine immunosuppressive regimens in cardiac transplantation: decreased hyperlipidemia and hypertension with tacrolimus. J Heart Lung Transplant 18: 336–345

Van Zee KJ, Kohno T, Fischer E, Rock CS, Moldawer LL, Lowry SF (1992) Tumor necrosis factor soluble receptors circulate during experimental and clinical inflammation and can protect against excessive tumor necrosis factor alpha in vitro and in vivo. Proc Natl Acad Sci USA 89: 4845–4849

Wallace CA (1998) The use of methotrexate in childhood rheumatic disease. Arthritis Rheum 41: 381–391

Wang Y, Calder VL, Lightman SL, Greenwood J (1995) Antigen presentation by rat brain and retinal endothelial cells. J Neuroimmunol 61: 231–239

Xiao BG, Link H (1997) Mucosal tolerance: a two-edged sword to prevent and treat autoimmune diseases. Clin Immunol Immunopathol 85: 119–128

Yang P, Das PK, Kijlstra A (2000) Localization and characterization of immunocompetent cells in the human retina. Ocul Immunol Inflamm 8: 149–157

Zhang J, Wu GS, Ishimoto S, Pararajasegaram G, Rao NA (1997) Expression of major histocompatibility complex molecules in rodent retina: immunohistochemical study. Invest Ophthalmol Vis Sci 38: 1848–1857

Advances in immunosuppressive treatment of juvenile idiopathic arthritis

Gerd Horneff*

Department of Pediatrics, Martin Luther University Halle-Wittenberg,
Halle, Federal Republic of Germany

Introduction

Autoimmune diseases tend to be less common in children than in adults, but incidences were not studied very well. Systemic autoimmune diseases, in particular, systemic lupus erythematosus (SLE), juvenile dermatomyositis, systemic sclerosis, primary and secondary vasculitis, sarcoidosis and inflammatory bowel disease do occur in childhood and require immunosuppressive treatment. Juvenile idiopathic arthritis is the most common systemic autoimmune disease and affects children of every age. During the first year of life, however, it is rare. The incidence is variable but about 10–20 per 100,000 and the prevalence is about 50–100 per 100,000 children below 16 years (Woo and Wedderburn 1998). The term juvenile idiopathic arthritis (JIA) has been raised in 1997 at the ILAR meeting (Petty et al. 1998) and will substitute for earlier terms like juvenile arthritis, juvenile rheumatoid arthritis (Brewer et al. 1977), and juvenile chronic arthritis (JCA). The diagnosis is given in children up to the age of 16 years with chronic arthritis persisting for at least 6 weeks when other possible causes of arthritis have been excluded. Subclassification into six groups has to be performed after a course of the disease of 6 months (Table 1).

This classification attempts to put together clinically homogeneous groups according to their clinical features at presentation and their disease progression. It will be a continuing process as genetics and disease mechanisms become known. Subclassification will enable better studies about the etiology, the pathogenesis as well as on treatment and prognosis. Similarities of all subgroups are the appearance of arthritis, morning stiffness and tenosynovitis as well as growth disturbance, which may lead to a minor or overgrowth of limbs or growth delay

* Author's address: Universitätsklinik und Poliklinik für Kinder- und Jugendmedizin, 06097 Halle, Federal Republic of Germany.
E-mail: gerd.horneff@medizin.uni-halle.de

Table 1. Classification of JIA

Subtype	Extraarticular manifestation
1 Systemic arthritis	Fever, evanescent skin rash, hepatomegaly, splenomegaly, pericarditis, pleuritis, lymphadenopathy, vasculitis, growth failure, dystrophy
2 Seronegative polyarthritis[a]	Low-grade fever, tenosynovitis, uveitis, vasculitis
3 Seropositive polyarthritis[a]	Low-grade fever, tenosynovitis, uveitis, vasculitis, rheumatoid nodules
4a Early-onset oligoarthritis[b]	Chronic uveitis
4b Extended oligoarthritis[c]	Chronic uveitis
5 Enthesitis-related arthritis	Enthesitis, acute uveitis
6 Psoriasis and arthritis	Psoriasis
7 Unclassified arthritis or criteria of more than one category are fulfilled	

[a] At least 5 joints are inflamed
[b] Maximal 4 inflamed joints
[c] Maximal 4 inflamed joints during the first 6 months of the disease followed by at least 5 inflamed joints thereafter

and dystrophy, especially in children with polyarticular subtype or systemic arthritis.

The prognosis depends on the subtype at presentation, defined by the number of affected joints and on accompanying extraarticular manifestations. The rate of mortality of earlier investigation tends to be about up to 4%, in later studies less than 1%. Children with systemic arthritis are much more at risk than others and may succumb of amyloidosis, cardiologic complications, macrophage activation syndrome and complications related to treatment (Wallace and Levinson 1991). 22–41% of children presenting with oligoarticular disease, 50% of children with polyarticular and 27–48% of children with systemic onset will have persisting active arthritis for at least 10 years (Petty 1999) with an inverse rate of remissions. Whether the actual advantage of therapeutic options will improve the prognosis, has to be the topic of future analysis.

Conventional drug treatment of JIA

Current treatment recommendations for JIA depend on the subtype and severity of the disease. In mild disease, treatment with nonsteroidal antirheumatics (NSAIDs) may be sufficient. Fever, organ involvement as well as severe disease will indicate the need of corticosteroids. Short-term toxicity is well known. However, long-term toxicity is a major concern and particular growth suppression is common. There were no treatment recommendations available how to use corticosteroids in JIA. Intraarticular steroid treatment is safe and effective, in many cases obviating the need for NSAID treatment. Treatment guidelines for the use of high-dose oral corticosteroids do exist in childhood nephrotic syndrome and in juvenile dermatomyositis. In idiopathic nephrotic syndrome, prednisone is given

Table 2. Reported applications of steroid pulse therapy

Systemic lupus erythematosus
Systemic sclerosis
Dermatomyositis (including juvenile DM[a])
Rheumatoid arthritis
Juvenile idiopathic arthritis
Glomerulonephritis
Immune thrombocytopenia
Cutaneous autoimmune diseases (pemphigus...)
Transplantation medicine

---

[a] Controlled study available in children

at a dosage of 60 mg/m^2 for 6 weeks followed by 40 mg/m^2 every second day for 6 weeks. In juvenile dermatomyositis 1–2 mg/kg of body weight is given for 4–8 weeks, followed by tapering of the dosage over 4–6 months if therapeutic success could be achieved. Pulsed intravenous methylprednisolone (30 mg/kg on 3 consecutive days) as an inducing agent is used for treatment of JIA by several centers and may have advantages over conventional steroid therapy since there were less side effects. The endogenous cortisone production is reduced by only 72 h, bone metabolism is only shortly inhibited and influence on growth is low if present at all. It has been used in a number of autoimmune or inflammatory diseases (Table 2). Additional side effects include nausea, psychosis, arterial hypertonus, arrhythmia and sudden death. Long-term use of corticosteroids is undesirable because of its multiple side effects and further studies are needed to find the best method of steroid treatment for JIA.

Disease-modifying drugs like gold salts, chloroquine, sulfasalazine or immunosuppressives may be indicated in persistent disease. However, there is no standard procedure when to start and what will be the first drug of choice. Methotrexate (MTX), sulfasalazine and azathioprine have been shown to be effective in at least one randomized placebo-controlled trial in JIA (Kvien et al. 1986, van Rossum et al. 1998, Giannini et al. 1992, Woo et al. 2000). Cyclosporine is used as a combinatory agent in resistant disease, especially in systemic JIA. However, there are too few data supporting these recommendations.

Azathioprine, a purine analogue metabolized to 6-mercaptopurine, interferes with the DNA synthesis by inhibition of purine synthesis. It is used in several childhood autoimmune diseases. Examples are SLE, dermatomyositis, Crohn's disease and autoimmune hepatitis. Adverse events include thrombocytopenia, leucopenia, anaemia and hepatic toxicity. Its cancerogenicity is still a matter of debate. In JIA there is only a single controlled study demonstrating a weak advantage of the drug over placebo (Kvien et al. 1986).

Sulfasalazine, an analogue of salicylic acid and sulfapyridine, has been introduced in the management of JIA. Its advantage is the relatively low toxicity. Adverse reactions are not necessarily minor, however, and gastrointestinal irritation, mucosal ulcerations, leucopenia, as well as severe muco-cutaneous reactions have been described. There are few publications on the use of sulfasalazine in JIA and only one controlled study, which shows a minor advantage over placebo (van Rossum et al. 1998).

Methotrexate has become a mainstay in the treatment of JIA. There were numerous open reports and two randomized placebo-controlled studies demonstrated its efficiency (Giannini et al. 1992, Woo et al. 2000). It is used also in other childhood autoimmune diseases, juvenile dermatomyositis, scleroderma and SLE. At the dosage of 10–15 mg/m^2 of body surface, it appears to be more anti-inflammatory than immunosuppressive. Resistant cases may respond to doses as high as 1 mg/kg. Since the absorption of oral methotrexate is limited, high doses have to be given parenterally. Subcutaneous injections are better tolerated, with similar absorption profiles to intramuscular injections (Brooks et al. 1990). Adverse effects limiting its availability are abdominal discomfort, nausea, vomiting, hepatotoxicity, leucopenia, anaemia, mucositis, and alopecia. Concern about long-term toxicity dealt with hepatic and lung fibrosis and interstitial pneumonitis. Because of its high teratogenic potential careful birth control has to be warranted.

Biologics for treatment of JIA

Etanercept

Tumor necrosis factor alpha (TNF-α) is a soluble 17 kDa protein consisting of 3 identical subunits and is mainly produced by T cells, monocytes and macrophages. Target cells express two specific receptors, a 55 kDa and a 75 kDa receptor. They were also found in a soluble form secreted into the plasma, neutralising superabundant TNF-α. By this way, the balance between proinflammatory and anti-inflammatory mediators is kept. Overexpression of proinflammatory cytokines IL-1 (interleukin-1), IL-6 and TNF-α has been shown in rheumatoid arthritis, JIA and other autoimmune inflammatory diseases and will overturn the balance (Fig. 1). Etanercept, a 75 kDa TNF receptor-Fcγ$_1$ fusion protein, binds TNF with high affinity and can interfere decisively in the cytokine cascade leading at the final point to inflammation and joint destruction. The cytokine cascade downstream of TNF-α will include IL-1 and IL-6 into the proinflammatory process (Fig. 2). Blocking of TNF therefore will in part also diminish effects of these cytokines.

Several studies in adults with rheumatoid arthritis have demonstrated a marked anti-inflammatory response to etanercept. A single placebo-controlled trial has been performed in children with polyarticular JIA (Lovell et al. 2000). 69 children, age between 4 and 17 years, suffering from polyarticular JIA who had resistant disease to a prior treatment with methotrexate or who have not tolerated methotrexate entered the study. 22 patients had systemic, 40 patients had polyarticular and 7 patients had oligoarticular onset of the disease. At least 4 active inflamed joints and 2 tender joints with limiting of motion were necessary for inclusion in the study. NSAIDs and a stable low dose of corticosteroids were allowed in parallel. At first, all children were treated with etanercept at a dosage of 0.4 mg/kg of body weight twice weekly for 3 months. 51 patients (74%) demonstrated improvement of at least 30% in 3 of 6 core set criteria for improvement of juvenile arthritis (Table 3).

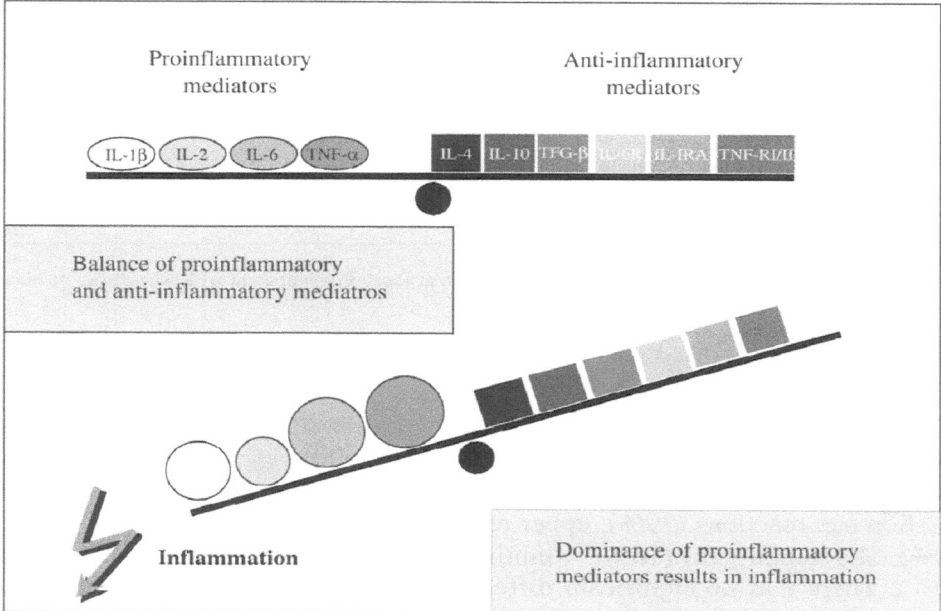

Fig. 1. Hypothesis 1: Control of inflammation is mediated by a balance of proinflammatory cytokines, IL-1, IL-3, IL-6, and TNF, and anti-inflammatory cytokines, cytokine antagonists and soluble receptors. Hypothesis 2: Inflammation will result from excess proinflammatory mediators

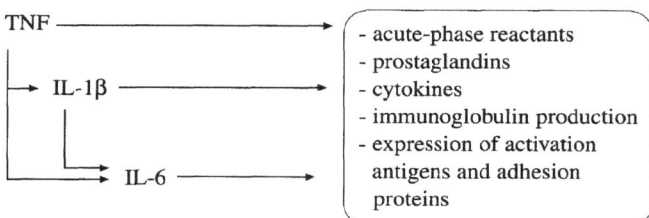

Fig. 2. TNF plays a central role in inflammation since it is able to enhance directly the production of acute-phase reactants, prostaglandins, immunoglobulins, the expression of activation antigens and adhesion proteins and in addition to induce IL-1 and IL-6 which themselves have pluripotent inflammatory activity. Blocking of TNF therefore diminishes not only TNF but also IL-1 and IL-6 activity

51 responders were capable for inclusion to the following placebo-controlled double-blind study for further 3 months, demonstrating clearly the superiority of etanercept over placebo. The number of patients achieving a 30% response rate or a 50% response rate was significantly higher in the treatment group (P < 0.001). Considerable improvement in all measures of disease activity was sustained in children on drug. Children treated with placebo demonstrated increasing numbers of active and tender joints, duration of morning stiffness and patient and physician's global assessment. In addition ESR (erythrocyte sedimentation rate) and

Table 3. Juvenile arthritis: core set criteria for improvement (Giannini et al. 1997)[a]

1. Physician's global assessment of the severity of the disease (10 cm visual analogue scale)
2. Global assessment of overall well being by the patient or parent (10 cm visual analogue scale)
3. Number of "active" joints (joints with swelling or joints with limiting of motion and with pain, tenderness or both)
4. Number of joints with limiting of motion
5. Functional score (Childhood Health Assessment Questionnaire)
6. Erythrocyte sedimentation rate

[a] Improvement is defined by decrease of at least 30% in at least 3 of 6 criteria with worsening of no more than one of the six response criteria for more than 30%

CRP (C-reactive protein) levels re-increased, while children receiving the active drug showed further improvement (Lovell et al. 2000).

Etanercept was safe and well tolerated. Only minor adverse events occurred: injection site reactions (39%), upper respiratory tract infections (35%), headache (20%), abdominal pain (16%), vomiting (14%), diarrhoea (12%), and skin rash (10%). There was no significant difference in the occurrence of adverse events between the control group and the treatment group. A generalised skin rash in 1 patient occurred after the first injection and led to exclusion from the study. This controlled study was followed by open trials and case studies demonstrating the therapeutic efficacy even in patients with so far refractory disease (Kietz et al. 2001).

JIA subtype and efficacy

Already the controlled trial showed that children with systemic arthritis demonstrated lesser efficacy than children with polyarticular or oligoarticular JIA (Lovell et al. 2000). 4 of 9 children (44%) with systemic arthritis developed a predefined disease flare upon treatment, but so did only 3 of 16 children with other subtypes. Analysis of etanercept treatment of 41 French JIA patients showed that 5 of 11 children with systemic arthritis but 11 of 12 children with other subtypes responded well to treatment with etanercept (Prieur et al. 2000). Unpublished data of the German registry for treatment of children with etanercept demonstrated that 10 of 37 (27%) patients with systemic JIA but only 1 of 103 (1%) patients with other subtypes discontinued therapy because of lack of efficacy. Therefore therapeutic efficacy is likely to be lower in children with systemic arthritis. This seems not to be dose related since higher doses of etanercept did not result in an increase in efficacy (Takei et al. 2001).

Long-term experience with etanercept in childhood

An open-label follow-up study was undertaken with 50 patients following the controlled trial (Lovell et al. 2001). Patients treated with etanercept during the initial open part and during the controlled part showed continuous therapeutic efficacy throughout the whole observation period of at least 2 years. Those who have been treated with placebo for 3 months demonstrated an equal therapeutic efficiency after entering the open label. After 2 years of treatment 78% of patients showed an improvement of at least 50% defined by the core set criteria. Tolerance was excellent. There were no autoimmune reactions, no SLE-like syndrome and no remarkable infections. Postmarketing studies are ongoing. In Germany a registry for children was set up to gain knowledge about the therapeutic efficiency, tolerability and safety of long-term administration of etanercept.

Infectious diseases are one major concern as it is for the use of other immunosuppressives. In a world-wide etanercept safety database over 103,000 mostly rheumatoid-arthritis patients were collected with 102,000 patient years of experience. The rate of serious infections observed in etanercept trials is 4.3 per 100 patient years with no increase in infections over time. This rate is within the range (3.9–12.8 per 100 patient years) previously described in the pre-TNF antagonist era (Wallis et al. 2001). Another concern is the development of autoimmune diseases or malignancies. There were a couple of reports of an SLE-like syndrome as well as demyelination diseases and anemia coming up on TNF antagonists. Insulin-dependent diabetes mellitus was observed in one child five months after starting etanercept. Albeit antibodies to glutamate decarboxylase were detectable in serum collected prior therapy, and coexistence of diabetes and JIA has been mentioned in the literature, treatment with etanercept could have anticipated the course of the diabetes (Bloom 2000), since there is at least one animal study showing a negative correlation between the levels of TNF and the occurrence of an insulin-dependent diabetes. Demyelination disease has been noted mainly in adults. However, there is also one report of demyelination in one child (Sicotte and Voskuhl 2001). Systematic registration of adverse effects in Germany collected several noninfectious adverse events, skin reactions, cutaneous vasculitis, headache, stomach ache and infectious events, herpes labialis, chickenpox, molluscs and one septic arthritis in a child receiving a joint puncture with injection of triamcinolone.

Opportunistic infections were mainly observed in adult patients treated with infliximab. This problem may be related to a different way of action and seems not to be that important in etanercept therapy.

Combination therapy with methotrexate

The safety and efficacy of etanercept plus methotrexate combination therapy has been demonstrated in a 6-month blinded trial in adults (Weinblatt et al. 1999). First experiences in children have been reported in open studies (Schmeling et al. 2001). Albeit several disease-modifying antirheumatic drugs including methotrexate have failed alone, combination therapy led to a rapid and sustained response in all 6 children. Morning stiffness and joint tenderness completely disappeared and 3 children were free of symptoms after 6 months of therapy. Long-term experience with combination therapy is now available of 14 patients with previously refractory JIA for 12 to 36 months and led to complete remission in 9 patients and partial remission with no tender joints and no morning stiffness in the remainders

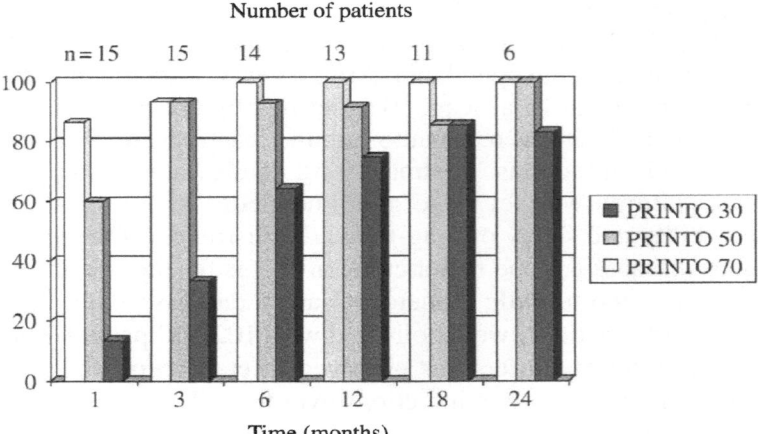

Fig. 3. Proportion of patients achieving a response according to the PRINTO criteria (Giannini et al. 1997): improvement of at least 3 of 6 core set criteria (Table 3) of 30, 50 or 70% respectively with worsening of no more than 1 criterion for more than 30%. Treatment was discontinued in the only 1 patient with systemic arthritis after 3 months because of inefficiency and after 12 months of therapy in 1 girl who developed recurrent uveitis while she was without any joint symptoms. One child was lost for follow up after 12 months of therapy

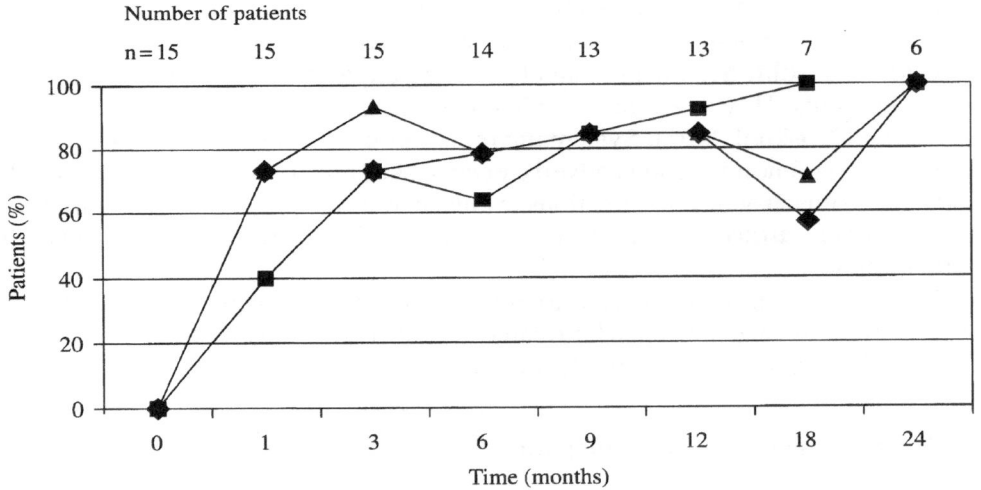

Fig. 4. Proportion of patients with normal levels of IL-6 (<5 pg/l, ■), CRP (<5 mg/l, ♦), and ESR (<10 mm/l, ▲) in response to treatment with etanercept and methotrexate

(Fig. 3). Most patients demonstrated normalization of ESR, CRP and serum levels of IL-6 (Fig. 4). Corticosteroids were discontinued in 10 patients and decreased by at least 50% in the others. Neither tapering down corticosteroids nor discontinuation of methotrexate led to a flare of the disease. Tolerability of combination therapy was good. However, 3 patients demonstrated liver enzyme abnormalities, which disappeared after discontinuation of methotrexate. In one child, recurrent uveitis occurred in a situation of complete rheumatological remission. Etanercept has been discontinued and a flare with active arthritis occurred 3 weeks later. Combination studies with other disease-modifying antirheumatic drugs have not been reported of children. Combination with sulfasalazine in some children led to leucopenia. Reduction in the dosage of sulfasalazine resulted in correction of the leucopenia in all cases (Striegel et al. 2001).

Etanercept and uveitis

Children with JIA are at high risk for the development of chronic uveitis. The therapeutic efficacy of etanercept for treatment of uveitis has been investigated in only one open trial. A significant drop in cellularity was observed in 10 of 16 affected eyes, and 4 of 18 eyes showed complete remission (Reiff et al. 2001). It is worth mentioning that there were several children developing uveitis upon treatment. In these patients however, treatment was not sufficient to prevent or treat uveitis. Therefore, the value of etanercept for treatment of chronic uveitis remains to be established.

Etanercept in juvenile ankylosing spondylitis

The use of TNF-targeting therapy has opened new perspectives for the treatment of ankylosing spondylitis. Controlled studies have been performed in adults with at first infliximab followed by etanercept (Brandt et al. 2000, Marzo-Ortega et al. 2001). Treatment of 8 patients with juvenile ankylosing spondylitis led to marked improvement in all patients with improvement of morning stiffness, decrease of the number of active joints and ESR and increase of hemoglobin levels (Reiff and Henrickson 2001). These results were comparable to results obtained in adults treated in randomized controlled studies.

Etanercept in periodic-fever syndromes

Children with systemic JIA typically present with spiking fever refractory to antibiotic treatment. Their prognosis is uncertain which in part is due to the heterogeneity of the disease. However, there are a couple of febrile diseases presenting with fever, skin reactions and arthritis and arthralgia. These include the familial mediterranean fever, a mutation in the pyrin/marenostrin gene, the periodic fever, aphthous stomatitis, pharyngitis and adenitis syndrome, the TNF-receptor-associated periodic fever syndrome, the hyper-IgD syndrome, the Muckle–Wells syndrome, familial cold urtikaria, and others. The TNF-receptor-associated periodic-fever syndrome is caused by a mutation of the 55 kDa TNF receptor leading to a defective shedding of the receptor. Therefore, soluble TNF cannot be neutralized, which leads to intensified and prolonged action of TNF via membrane-bound p55 or p75 TNF receptors. This results in a clinically distinct disease with periodic fever lasting days to weeks, arthralgia, myalgia and serositis which can be misdiagnosed as systemic JIA. Efficacy of TNF antagonism is likely explained by neutralization of the TNF excess. In a study enrolling 15 children with known mutations in the TNF-R gene, treatment with etanercept for a 3-month period resulted in a significant decrease of symptoms compared to the period directly before and after treatment. Patient's symptoms returned to pretreatment symptom levels following the withdrawal of etanercept. Similarly, etanercept was shown to dose-dependently decrease the baseline CRP, ESR, and the amount of NSAIDs and corticosteroids used (Hull et al. 2001). The hyper-IgD syndrome, a variant of mevalone aciduria is also characterized by periodic fever, arthritis, rash and serositis. Etanercept seems to have beneficial effects in this disease too (Takada et al. 2001). Since these diseases are very rare, controlled studies will not be possible before recommendation for treatment.

Infliximab

Infliximab is a murine-human chimeric monoclonal antibody against TNF-α that is approved for the treatment of rheumatoid arthritis and Crohn's disease. Its efficacy has been shown in randomized controlled trials in adults with rheumatoid arthritis either in single-drug therapy or in combination therapy with methotrexate (Maini et al. 1999). However, infections are a major concern. Especially reactivation of tuberculosis may develop soon after initiation of therapy (Keane et al. 2001). Experience with infliximab in JIA is very limited. There were case studies and open reports. In one cohort of JIA patients with so far refractory disease, infusions of 3 mg of infliximab per kg of body weight every 4 weeks resulted in a marked decrease of the number of active joints, ESR and levels of CRP (Gerloni et al. 2000). One patient unsuccessfully treated previously with etanercept also improved. 4 children with systemic JIA refractory to a standard-dose infliximab therapy have been treated with higher doses up to 20 mg/kg. All patients responded, indicating the importance of dose-finding studies which have not been performed in children neither for infliximab nor for etanercept (Kiamura et al. 2001).

Further cytokines and cytokine antagonists

The recombinant soluble IL-1 receptor antagonist (IL1RA) anakinra has been approved for treatment of rheumatoid arthritis in the U.S.A. IL-1RA binds to the IL-1 receptor without intrinsic activity and is by this way blocking IL-1 function. Anti-inflammatory and clinical effects were less pronounced than those seen by TNF-blocking agents. Radiological progression however is markedly diminished (Jiang et al. 2000). There were no studies in children so far.

Antibodies to IL-6 have been tried in very early studies in adults with rheumatoid arthritis but failed to have sustained clinical effects, possibly due to a prolongation of the half-life of biologically active antibody-bound IL-6 in the plasma. Anti-IL-6 receptor antibodies, blocking the binding of IL-6 to its receptor, however were shown to have anti-inflammatory effects. Open studies in adults demonstrated clinical efficacy comparable to the TNF blockers. Anti-inflammatory cytokines, IL-4 and IL-10, are future candidates for an immunologically based therapy; as well as beta interferon subtype 1a, which shows anti-inflammatory activity on T-cells in vitro. Clinical usefulness has been shown in a preliminary open study in 6 children with active JIA refractory to methotrexate. All patients demonstrated an at least 30% improvement of the core set criteria and 3 showed a 50% improvement. In patients with systemic arthritis, however, fever persisted (Sundel et al. 2001).

Thalidomide, best known because of its teratogenic effects, has inhibitory effects on proinflammatory cytokines including TNF and stimulates the production of anti-inflammatory cytokines, alpha interferon and IL-10. The use of the drug will further be limited because of its neurotoxic effects. 5 children with so far refractory systemic JIA, experienced with methotrexate, cyclosporine and etanercept, demonstrated improvement of clinical and laboratory disease activity parameters (Lehman et al. 2001). Therefore, cytokine-targeting therapies in the future using low-molecular-weight drugs will be possible. Other substances potentially interfering with the regulation of TNF production or the signal transduction pathway are awaiting.

Closing remarks

Current experience using TNF-blocking agents in childhood is very limited. However, marked clinical effects can be reached even in children with so far intractable disease. Furthermore, the velocity and the strength of its effects on clinical activity are remarkable. The influence on radiological progression has not been evaluated in children so far. Etanercept is the only biological agent approved for treatment of children with an age of at least 4 years who showed refractory and active disease. Current recommendations for treatment are noteworthy (Horneff et al. 2000). However, they are based not very much on experience but on theoretical considerations. Too little experience has been made with common situations in childhood like infections or vaccinations with live attenuated germs, which therefore should not be applied. Poor knowledge exists about combination therapy. So far, combination with methotrexate seems to be possible and meaningful but also risky at least with respect to infections. Other immunosuppressives should not be used for combinations. If TNF-blocking agents are considered, all children should carefully be investigated and monitored throughout treatment. Attention should be directed not only to infectious diseases but also to autoimmune diseases including "lupus-like syndrome", demyelination, diabetes mellitus and uveitis.

Interruption of therapy is mandatory in the case of severe infections and can be recommended before surgery. There is no reason for concern about a decrease of efficacy when the drug is reintroduced compared to the initial treatment. This has been clearly shown by the follow-up study performed after the controlled trial. Here already, there was no difference in treatment efficacy in children in whom etanercept was reintroduced after a 3-month placebo phase compared to those treated with etanercept throughout the study (Lovell et al. 2001). Prolonged discontinuation however can lead to a disease flare evident a few weeks later. Until now, there is no systematic study on what happens after discontinuation of TNF-blocking agents.

Modern immunologically based therapy coming from experiences with adults will frequently and rapidly be tried in children too. Albeit the biologic agents, notably the TNF inhibitors, have effected dramatic improvement in many children with severe disease who previously were often significantly disabled, studies in children remain of critical importance before recommending these agents for routine therapy. Today, without previous studies on efficacy and safety numerous drugs are used for treatment particular in severely ill children. This remains to be an unacceptable situation.

References

Bloom BJ (2000) Development of diabetes mellitus during etanercept therapy in a child with systemic onset juvenile rheumatoid arthritis. Arthritis Rheum 43: 2606–2608

Brandt J, Haibel H, Cornely D, Golder W, Gonzalez J, Reddig J, Thriene W, Sieper J, Braun J (2000) Successful treatment of active ankylosing spondylitis with the anti-tumor necrosis factor alpha monoclonal antibody infliximab. Arthritis Rheum 43: 1346–1352

Brewer EJ Jr, Bass J, Baum J, Cassidy JT, Fink C, Jacobs J, Hanson V, Levinson JE, Schaller J, Stillman JS (1977) Current proposed revision of JRA criteria: JRA Criteria Subcommittee of the Diagnostic and Therapeutic Criteria Committee of the American Rheumatism Section of the Arthritis Foundation. Arthritis Rheum 20 Suppl: 195–199

Brooks PJ, Spruil WJ, Parish RC, Birchmore DA (1990) Pharmacokinetics of methotrexate administered by intramuscular and subcutaneous injections in patients with rheumatoid arthritis. Arthritis Rheum 33: 91–94

Gerloni V, Pontikaki I, Desiati DF, Lupi E, Gattinara M, Fantini F (2000) Infliximab in the treatment of persistently active juvenile idiopathic (chronic) arthritis. Ann Rheum Dis 59: 741

Gianninni EH, Brewer EJ, Kuzmina N, et al (1992) Methotrexate in resistant juvenile rheumatoid arthritis: results of the U.S.A.-U.S.S.R. double blind, placebo-controlled trial. N Engl J Med 326: 1043–1049

Giannini EH, Ruperto N, Raveli A, Lovell DJ, Felson DT, Martini A (1997) Preliminary definition of improvement in juvenile arthritis. Arthritis Rheum 40: 1202–1209

Horneff G, Forster J, Seyberth W, Michels H (2001) Empfehlungen der Arbeitsgemeinschaft Kinder- und Jugendrheumatologie zur Therapie mit Etanercept (P75 TNF-Rezeptor-Immunglobulinfusionsprotein). Z Rheumatol 59: 365–369

Hull K, Dean JA, Singh H, O'Shea JJ, Kastner DL (2001) Effect of Etanercept in the treatment of TNF-receptor associated periodic fever syndrome (TRAPS). Arthritis Rheum 44: 124S

Jiang Y, Genant HK, Watt I, Cobby M, Bresnihan B, Aitchison R, McCabe D (2000) A multicenter, double-blind, dose-ranging, randomized, placebo-controlled study of recombinant human interleukin-1 receptor antagonist in patients with rheumatoid arthritis: radiologic progression and correlation of Genant and Larsen scores. Arthritis Rheum 43: 1001–1009

Keane J, Gershon S, Wise RP, Mirabile-Levens E, Kasznica J, Schwieterman WD, Siegel JN, Braun MM (2001) Tuberculosis associated with infliximab, a tumor necrosis factor alpha-neutralizing agent. N Engl J Med 345: 1098–1104

Kietz DA, Permuelller PH, Moore TL (2001) Clinical response to Etanercept in polyarticular course juvenile rheumatoid arthritis. J Rheumatol 28: 360–362

Kimura Y, Imundo LF, Li SC (2001) High dose infliximab in the treatment of resistant systemic JRA. Arthritis Rheum 44: 272S

Kvien TK, Hoyeraal HM, Sandstad B (1986) Azathioprine versus placebo in patients with juvenile rheumatoid arthritis: a single center double blind comparative study. J Rheumatol 13: 118–123

Lehman TJA, Striegel KH, Onel KB (2001) Thalimomide therapy for corticosteroid dependent systemic onset juvenile rheumatoid arthritis. Arthritis Rheum 44: 272S

Lovell DJ, Giannini EH, Lange M, Burge DJ, Finck BK (1991) Sustained safety and efficacy of etanercept (enbrel) in the extended treatment of polyarticular-course JRA. Ann Rheum Dis Suppl 11: ii12

Lovell DJ, Giannini EH, Reiff A et al (2000) Etanercept in children with polyarticular juvenile rheumatoid arthritis. N Engl J Med 342: 763–769

Maini R, St Clair EW, Breedveld F, Furst D, Kalden J, Weisman M, Smolen J, Emery P, Harriman G, Feldmann M, Lipsky P (1999) Infliximab (chimeric anti-tumour necrosis factor alpha monoclonal antibody) versus placebo in rheumatoid arthritis patients receiving concomitant methotrexate: a randomised phase III trial. ATTRACT Study Group. Lancet 354: 1932–1939

Marzo-Ortega H, McGonagle D, O'Connor P, Emery P (2001) Efficacy of etanercept in the treatment of the entheseal pathology in resistant spondylarthropathy: a clinical and magnetic resonance imaging study. Arthritis Rheum 44: 2112–2117

Petty RE (1999) Prognosis in children with rheumatic diseases: justification for consideration of new therapies. Rheumatology (Oxford) 38: 739–742

Petty RE, Southwood TR, Baum J et al (1998) Revision of the proposed criteria for juvenile idiopathic arthritis: Durban 1997. J Rheumatol 25: 1991–1994

Prieur AM, Mouy R, Debré M, Quatrier P (2000) French Enbrel Registry. Pres Meeting 2000 Abstract. Ann Rheum Dis 59: 745

Reiff A, Henrickson M (2001) Prolonged efficacy of etanercept in refractory juvenile ankylosing spondylitis. Arthritis Rheum 44: 292S

Reiff A, Takei S, Sadeghi S, Stout A, Shaham B, Bernstein B, Gallagher K, Stout T (2001) Etanercept therapy in children with treatment-resistant uveitis. Arthritis Rheum 44: 1411–1415

Schmeling H, Mathony K, John V, Keyßer G, Burdach S, Horneff G (2001) Combination of etanercept and methotrexate for the treatment of refractory juvenile idiopathic arthritis: a pilot study. Ann Rheum Dis 60: 410–412

Sicotte NL, Voskuhl RR (2001) Onset of multiple sclerosis associated with anti-TNF therapy. Neurology 57: 1885–1888

Striegel KH, Onel KB, Thomas J, Lehman TJA (2001) Leukopenia in children receiving sulfasalazine and etanercept. Arthritis Rheum 44: 292S

Sundel RP, Wallace CA, Zurakowski A (2001) Pilot trial of Interferon β1a (Avonex®) in JRA. Arthritis Rheum 44: 272S

Takada K, Aksentijevich I, Kelley RI, Kastner DL (2001) Effect of Etanercept therapy in a child with hyper-IgD and periodic fever syndrome (HIDS). Arthritis Rheum 44: 124S

Takei S, Groh D, Bernstein B, Shaham B, Gallagher K, Reiff A (2001) Safety and efficacy of high dose Etanercept in treatment of juvenile rheumatoid arthritis. J Rheumatol 28: 1677–1680

Van Rossum MAJ, Fiselier TJW, Frassen MJAM, et al (1998) Sulfasalzin in the treatment of juvenile chronic arthritis: a randomized double-blind placebo-controlled multicenter study. Arthritis Rheum 41: 808–816

Wallace CA, Levinson LE (1991) Juvenile rheumatoid arthritis: outcome and treatment for the 1990s. Rheum Dis Clin North Am 17: 891–905

Wallis WJ, Burge DJ, Sabath D, Gardiner M (2001) Tuberculosis reports with etanercept (Enbrel) therapy. Arthritis Rheum 44: 78S

Weinblatt ME, Kremer JM, Bankhurst C, Bulpitt KJ, Fleischmann RM, Fox RI, et al (1999) A trial of etanercept, a recombinant tumor necrosis factor receptos:Fc fusion protein, in patients with rheumatic arthritis. N Engl J Med 340: 253–259

Woo P, Wedderburn RL (1998) Juvenile chronic arthritis. Lancet 351: 969–973

Woo P, Southwood TR, Prieur AM, Dore CJ, Grainger J, David J, Ryder C, Hasson N, Hall A, Lemelle I (2000) Randomized, placebo-controlled, crossover trial of low-dose oral methotrexate in children with extended oligoarticular or systemic arthritis. Arthritis Rheum 43: 1849–1857

Significance of γδ T lymphocytes in autoimmune diseases

Dieter Kabelitz*

Institute of Immunology, University of Kiel, Federal Republic of Germany

Introduction

T lymphocytes are the effector cells of adaptive (or "specific") cellular immune responses. They recognize antigen via their heterodimeric T cell receptor (TCR) molecule which is non-covalently associated with the CD3 molecular complex on the surface of T cells. While the vast majority of mature T cells carries a "conventional" TCR composed of α and β chains, a small subset of T lymphocytes expresses the alternative γδ T cell receptor. γδ T cells usually account for 1–5% of peripheral blood T cells but are enriched in other anatomical localizations such as the intestine, where they constitute a major population within the intraepithelial T lymphocytes. A representative two-color flow cytometry dot plot analysis of αβ and γδ T lymphocytes in the peripheral blood of a healthy individual is shown in Fig. 1.

αβ T cells express CD4 or CD8 molecules, which are important coreceptors for major histocompatibility complex(MHC)-encoded antigens. αβ T cells thus recognize antigen in the form of processed peptides in association with MHC class II (for CD4$^+$ T cells) or MHC class I molecules (for CD8$^+$ T cells). In striking contrast, most γδ T lymphocytes lack CD4 and CD8 expression. Moreover, γδ T cells usually do not recognize MHC-associated peptides, but rather various stress-inducible cell surface molecules as well as low-molecular-weight metabolites that are secreted by certain bacteria and other microorganisms. In line with the lack of CD4 and CD8 expression, most γδ T cells are not MHC-restricted in their ligand recognition. In functional terms, γδ T cells share many features with αβ T lymphocytes. γδ T cells thus display potent cytotoxic activity and are capable of secreting a large array of different cytokines and chemokines. Several recent reviews have covered the features and functions of murine and human γδ T cells in great detail, and the reader is referred to these reviews for in-depth information

* Author's address: Institute of Immunology, University of Kiel, Michaelisstrasse 5, 24105 Kiel, Federal Republic of Germany.
E-mail: kabelitz@immunologie.uni-kiel.de

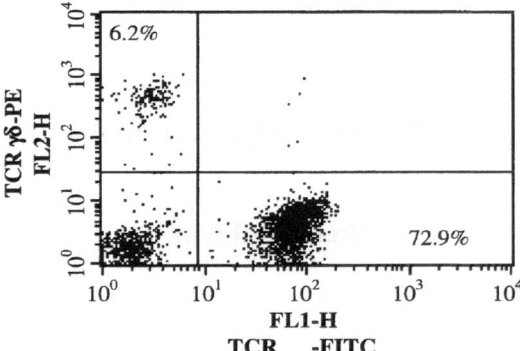

Fig. 1. αβ and γδ T lymphocytes in peripheral blood. Peripheral blood mononuclear cells isolated from a healthy adult individual were stained with fluorescein isothiocyanate-conjugated pan-αβ (BMA031; Cβ-specific; x-axis) and pan-γδ (TCRδ1; Cδ-specific; y-axis) monoclonal antibodies. Analysis was performed on a FACScan flow cytometer

Table 1. Major features of peripheral blood αβ and γδ T lymphocytes

Characteristic	αβ T lymphocytes	γδ T lymphocytes
Frequency	ca. 95%	ca. 5%
TCR germline repertoire	large (approximately 50 Vα, 50 Vβ genes)	small (6 Vγ, 6 Vδ genes)
CD4 and CD4 expression	60% CD4$^+$	<5% CD4$^+$
	30% CD8$^+$	ca. 20% CD8$^+$
	<2% CD4$^+$CD8$^+$	<1% CD4$^+$CD8$^+$
	<2% CD4$^-$CD8$^-$	ca. 80% CD4$^-$CD8$^-$
MHC restriction	CD4$^+$: MHC class II	most γδ T cells are not MHC restricted
	CD8$^+$: MHC class I	

(Chien and Hampl 2000, Hayday 2000, Kabelitz et al. 2000, Morita et al. 2000). A summary of the major differences between human αβ and γδ T lymphocytes is given in Table 1.

In the following sections, I will briefly review the basic differences between αβ and γδ T lymphocytes with respect to the TCR repertoire and the antigens recognized by the respective subpopulations. This will be followed by a discussion of the potential role of γδ T cells in autoimmunity.

T cell receptor repertoire of human γδ T lymphocytes

The conventional αβ T lymphocytes can recognize a seemingly unlimited variety of antigens in the form of short peptides generated from exogenous (e.g., bacterial) or endogenous (e.g., viral) antigens and presented to the αβ T cells in the context of MHC class II or class I molecules, respectively. The structural basis for the TCR repertoire resides in the process of the rearrangement of TCR genes that occurs during the intrathymic development and maturation of T lymphocyte precursors. A large number (approximately 50) of variable (V) gene segments encoding for Vα and Vβ elements is available in the germline genome, from which Vα/Vβ genes can be selected (Arden et al. 1995). In striking contrast, there are only six expressed human Vγ elements and a similarly small number of Vδ genes (Arden et al. 1995, Porcelli et al. 1991). Five of the expressed Vγ genes are closely related and, therefore, are grouped into the VγI family (Vγ 2, 3, 4, 5, 8), while Vγ9 is a single member of the VγII family (Porcelli et al. 1991). During recent years, monoclonal antibodies have been developed which allow to monitor the complete expressed human TCR Vγ repertoire by flow cytometry (Hinz et al. 1997). Interestingly, the few available TCR Vγ and Vδ genes are not randomly used. In the peripheral blood of healthy adults, there is a remarkable predominance of γδ T cells that specifically express Vγ9 in association with Vδ2, which can account for >90% of peripheral blood γδ T cells in individual donors (Wesch et al. 1998). Alterations in the TCR repertoire of peripheral blood γδ T cells are observed in certain diseases, notably HIV infection, where Vγ9Vδ2 cells are reduced and Vδ1-expressing γδ T cells usually predominate (Hinz et al. 1994, Wesch et al. 1998, Kabelitz et al. 1999). The predominance of Vγ9Vδ2-expressing cells within the peripheral blood γδ T cells of healthy individuals gradually develops during childhood and is thought to be due to the continuous exposure to γδ-stimulating environmental and/or microbial antigens (Parker et al. 1990). In contrast to peripheral blood, γδ T cells expressing Vδ1 in association with various Vγ elements are the major T cell population within the intraepithelial lymphocytes in the small intestine (Deusch et al. 1991). While the germline TCR Vγ/Vδ repertoire is small, the expressed repertoire is significantly enlarged by non-germline-encoded mechanisms such as the insertion of N nucleotides during gene rearrangement.

Ligands recognized by γδ T lymphocytes

αβ T cells recognize peptides presented on the surface of antigen-presenting cells such as dendritic cells or macrophages in the peptide-binding pocket of MHC class II or class I molecules. In contrast, peptide-specific MHC-restricted antigen recognition is rare among γδ T lymphocytes. Although peptide-specific murine γδ T cells have been identified (Born et al. 1990), this reactivity pattern is not representative of the majority of γδ T lymphocytes. Most studies of the specificity of murine γδ T cells have been performed with T cell hybridomas. At the clonal level, it has been shown that murine γδ T cells recognize MHC class II molecules IE independently of peptide and intracellular antigen presentation (Schild et al. 1994). γδ T cells also recognize nonclassical MHC class I-related molecules, some of which are inducible on activated or stressed cells. While the closely related MHC class Ib gene products T10 and T22 are recognized by murine γδ TCR (Bonneville et al. 1989, Weintraub et al. 1994), human γδ T cells expressing the Vδ1 element recognize the stress-inducible MHC class I-related MICA and MICB antigens (Groh et al. 1998). These findings together with the observation that murine skin-associated γδ T cells respond in a TCR-dependent fashion to heat-treated ("shocked") keratinocytes (Havran et al. 1991) support a scenario where γδ T lymphocytes play an indispensable role in the local immune surveillance against "stressed" epithelial cells. Moreover, members of the non-MHC-encoded but structurally related CD1 protein family can present self lipid antigens to human γδ T cells (Morita et al. 2000, Spada et al. 2000). One of the essential functions of T lymphocytes is the elimination of virus-infected cells. Cytotoxic CD8⁺ αβ T cells recognize viral peptides in the context of MHC class I molecules. In contrast, subsets of murine and human γδ T cells can recognize viral proteins without the requirement of MHC-dependent antigen presentation (Déchanet et al. 1999, Sciammas et al. 1994). Thus, it appears that there are fundamental differences in the pathway of antigen recognition between the αβ and the γδ TCR (Allison et al. 2001).

A large body of evidence indicates that γδ T lymphocytes are involved in the immune defense against infection. This evidence stems from the analysis of the role of γδ T cells in experimental models of infection (for a review, see Hayday 2000) and from the observation of a transient increase in γδ T cells in humans during the acute phase of several infectious diseases (for a review, see Kabelitz et al. 1999). Human γδ T cells expressing Vγ9 paired with Vδ2 respond to stimulation with *Mycobacterium tuberculosis* (Kabelitz et al. 1991). The mycobacterial ligands that are recognized by human γδ T cells have been characterized as phosphorylated low-molecular-weight nonproteinaceous molecules ("phosphoantigens"). Recently, the structure of several bacteria-derived phosphoantigens has been reported. Among the most potent γδ-activating ligands are bacterial metabolites derived from the non-mevalonate (or Rohmer) pathway of isoprenoid biosynthesis (Belmant et al. 1999, Morita et al. 2000, Altincicek et al. 2001). Such phosphoantigens are produced in large quantity by bacteria that lack the mevalonate pathway present in eukaryotic cells and they specifically target the dominant subset of Vγ9Vδ2-expressing human γδ T cells. In addition, the same subset of human γδ T cells is also activated by alkylamines derived from bacteria and certain plants (Bukowski et al. 1999). Taken together, it is quite clear that the majority of γδ T lymphocytes via their γδ TCR recognize ligands that are not seen by αβ T cells or any other cells in the immune system. A summary of the most frequent ligands for the γδ TCR is given in Table 2.

Table 2. Ligands recognized by γδ T lymphocytes

Murine γδ T cells	Human γδ T cells[a]
MHC class II (IE) without peptide	MHC class I-related MICA/MICB (Vδ1)
MHC class Ib antigens T10, T22	CD1c (Vδ1)
Herpes simplex virus glycoprotein I	Cytomegalovirus protein (mostly Vδ1)
Heat shock proteins	Low-molecular-weight molecules (Vγ9Vδ2):
	phosphoantigens
	alkylamines
	biphosphonates

[a] The TCR Vγ/Vδ usage of the responsive human γδ T cells is indicated in brackets; see Hayday (2000) for details

γδ T lymphocytes as effector cells of autoimmune disease

Given that γδ T cells can respond to potential self-antigens such as MHC class I-related antigens, CD1 molecules and heat shock proteins, it can be anticipated that γδ T cells might exert self-reactivity under certain circumstances and thereby contribute to autoimmune disease (Hayday and Geng 1997). In fact, it appears that some γδ T cells possess significant self-reactivity which is under stringent control of killer inhibitory receptors (KIR). KIR are cell surface receptors for MHC class I molecules which deliver inhibitory signals upon interaction with the corresponding MHC class I antigens. KIR of the heterodimeric CD94/NKG2A type are expressed on human Vγ9Vδ2 γδ T cells and control their reactivity pattern. If the interaction between the KIR and the relevant MHC class I antigens is blocked, TCR-dependent recognition of ligands expressed on autologous activated T lymphocytes is readily revealed in Vγ9Vδ2 cells, indicating stringent control of self-reactivity in this γδ T cell subset (Halary et al. 1997). Despite the obvious potential for self-reactivity of γδ T cells, there are only a few examples of autoimmune diseases resulting from γδ T cell-mediated autoreactivity (Yin and Craft 2000). Perhaps one of the best documented clinical examples is the case of a polymyositis mediated by a clonal population of human Vγ3Vδ2 γδ T cells (Hohlfeld et al. 1991, Pluschke et al. 1992). Unfortunately, the suspected auto-antigen has not been identified in these studies. A role of autoreactive γδ T cells was also suggested to contribute to the pathogenesis of multiple sclerosis. Here, it was found that γδ T cells isolated from the cerebrospinal fluid of multiple sclerosis patients killed oligodendrocytes via perforin- and Fas/CD95-dependent mechanisms (Zeine et al. 1998). Again, the ligands recognized by the cytotoxic γδ T cells were not identified. However, the colocalization of γδ T cells and heat shock protein 65-expressing oligodendrocytes suggests the possibility that heat shock protein might be involved (Selmaj et al. 1991). Moreover, the Vγ9Vδ2 T cells present in patients with multiple sclerosis are activated and can be induced to secrete high levels of proinflammatory cytokines, pointing again to a role of these cells in demyelinating diseases (Borsellino et al. 2000). Coeliac disease is yet another example of an autoimmune disease where characteristic alterations in the γδ T cell compartment occur. Coeliac disease is characterized by an allergy towards wheat proteins which is associated with autoimmunity directed towards tissue transglutaminase. An increase in the frequency of γδ T cells expressing a restricted TCR repertoire within the intraepithelial intestinal T cells is a characteristic feature of coeliac disease (Halstensen et al. 1989). Thus, alterations in the frequency and/or TCR repertoire of γδ T lymphocytes have been observed in several autoimmune diseases, notably rheumatoid arthritis (Keystone et al. 1991), autoimmune liver diseases (Martins et al. 1996), coeliac disease, and multiple sclerosis (for recent surveys, see Kabelitz et al. 1999, de Libero 2000). It should be emphasized, however, that these studies generally have not provided evidence for a direct involvement of γδ T cells as autoaggressive effector cells in autoimmune disease. It is more likely that changes in the γδ T cell compartment reflect a disturbance of a regulatory activity of γδ T cells in such diseases.

Regulatory role of γδ T lymphocytes in autoimmunity

In fact, substantial evidence supports the notion that γδ T cells regulate the auto-reactivity of other T lymphocyte populations and – directly or indirectly via T helper cells – the activity of autoantibody-producing B lymphocytes (Rajagopalan et al. 1990). Only a few examples can be discussed here. For a more comprehensive discussion of this topic, the reader is referred to recent reviews (Hayday and Geng 1997, Yin and Craft 2000). Several experimental strategies such as the deletion of γδ T cells by homologous recombination or the depletion by antibody treat-ment, as well as cell transfer experiments, have been used to address the issue of a regulatory role of γδ T cells. Peng and coworkers have crossed the lupus-prone MRL/Mp-*lpr/lpr* mice (which have a defect in the Fas/CD95 gene) with TCRβ$^{-/-}$ or TCRδ$^{-/-}$ mice (i.e., mice which lack αβ or γδ T cells). They observed that the *lpr* mice lacking γδ T cells developed higher titers of autoantibodies and suffered from more severe immune complex deposition in the glomeruli of the kidney and increased mortality as compared to the control *lpr* mice. Conversely, αβ T cell-deficient *lpr* mice developed a partial lupus syndrome with isotype-specific hyper-gammaglobulinemia and mild immune complex renal disease, which resulted from γδ-T-cell-dependent B cell help. From this data the authors concluded that γδ T cells participated both in the regulation and the propagation of murine lupus (Peng et al. 1996). Rajan and coworkers used depletion by antibody treatment to investigate the role of γδ T cells in a murine model of experimental allergic encephalomyelitis. They showed that the depletion of γδ T cells immediately before the onset of disease ameliorated the clinical severity of experimental aller-gic encephalomyelitis. More specifically, they demonstrated that the depletion of γδ T cells resulted in a dramatically reduced expression of proinflammatory cytokines IL-1 and IL-6 in the spinal cord, together with a marked reduction in cellular infiltrates, suggesting that γδ T cells regulated the influx of inflammatory cells and the levels of proinflammatory cytokines in the spinal cord (Rajan et al. 1998). On the basis of the substantial evidence for a regulatory role of γδ T cells in the immune network, attempts to explore the potential therapeutical capacity of regulatory γδ T cells have been initiated. In various experimental models, regu-latory γδ T cells have been induced by exposure to the relevant autoantigen through aerosol inhalation or oral application. An impressive example is the regu-lation of insulin-dependent diabetes in the nonobese diabetic NOD mouse model. The pancreatic pathology and the incidence of diabetes can be significantly reduced by the aerosol application of insulin after the onset of subclinical disease. Splenocytes of insulin-treated mice can suppress the adoptive transfer of diabetes to nondiabetic mice by T lymphocytes of diabetic mice. Harrison and coworkers successfully identified the nature of this regulatory cell as a CD8$^+$ splenic γδ T cell. The transfer of small numbers (in the order of 10^5) of CD8$^+$ γδ T cells from the spleen of insulin aerosol-treated NOD mice prevented diabetes in irradiated nondiabetic NOD mice which had received 2×10^7 splenocytes from overtly diabetic (i.e., old) NOD mice (Harrison et al. 1996). Interestingly, such regulatory γδ T cells can be also induced by oral administration of the relevant autoantigen. In Lewis rats, an αβ-T-cell-mediated experimental autoimmune uveitis is triggered by the subcutaneous immunization with a peptide of the retinal soluble antigen (S-antigen). In this experimental model, autoimmune uveitis can be prevented by transfer of γδ T cells from rats orally tolerized with the same S-antigen peptide (Wildner et al. 1996). Interestingly enough, the suppressive γδ T cell population identified in the studies by Wildner and coworkers displayed specificity for the 14-amino-acid S-antigen peptide which was used for oral induction, as shown by a proliferative response to the peptide in the presence of irradiated αβ T cells as antigen-presenting cells. Unfortunately, the mechanism of the suppressor activity of γδ T cells in these experimental models has not yet been precisely defined and requires further investigation. It is likely that the secretion of inhibitory cytokines such as IL-10 contributes to the suppressor activity of regulatory γδ T cells induced by oral or aerosol application of autoantigens (Hanninen and Harrison 2000). Interestingly, γδ T cell proliferation in response to activated autologous αβ T cell clones was observed in multiple sclerosis patients following vaccination with myelin basic protein-reactive T lymphocytes. The in vitro activated γδ T cells displayed low cytotoxic reactivity towards the vaccine αβ T cell clones but produced high levels of cytokines including IL-10 (Stinissen et al. 1998). Taken together, it appears that the regulatory activity of γδ T cells is mediated at least in part by the production of inhibitory cytokines.

Concluding remarks

Even after more than 15 years of research, the significance of γδ T cells is still under debate. It appears that some functions of γδ T cells are unique to this cell population, and others might be shared with other cells of the immune system. In this regard, γδ T cells might be considered as a link between the specific (or adaptive) and the nonspecific (or innate) immune system (Fig. 2).

Among the unique features of γδ T cells are the selective reactivity of a dominant γδ T cell subset to microbial danger signals such as phosphorylated intermediates derived from bacteria-specific metabolic pathways and the reactivity towards stress-induced MHC class I-related molecules. The latter observation suggests that γδ T cells might play a critical role in the local immune surveillance, a notion that is supported by the finding that dendritic epidermal γδ T cells can produce keratinocyte growth factor, thereby contributing to tissue repair (Boismenu and Havran 1994). Moreover, γδ T cells are also important in the regulation of cellular homeostasis in the intestine. The development of crypt intestinal epithelial cells is thus drastically disturbed in γδ knock-out (TCRδ$^{-/-}$) mice (Komano et al. 1995). Apart from the recognition of ligands which are not seen by any other cells of the immune system, γδ T cells also exert regulatory activities. Most impressive are the well-documented examples of transferable suppressor activity of γδ T cells, of which a few examples have been discussed above. While the term suppressor cell has been avoided in recent years, the discovery of CD25^{+}-regulatory αβ T cells (Shevach 2000) has raised new interest in the molecular characterization of suppressor mechanisms. Given the potent regulatory activity of γδ T cells in experimental animal models, it is certainly of major interest to explore

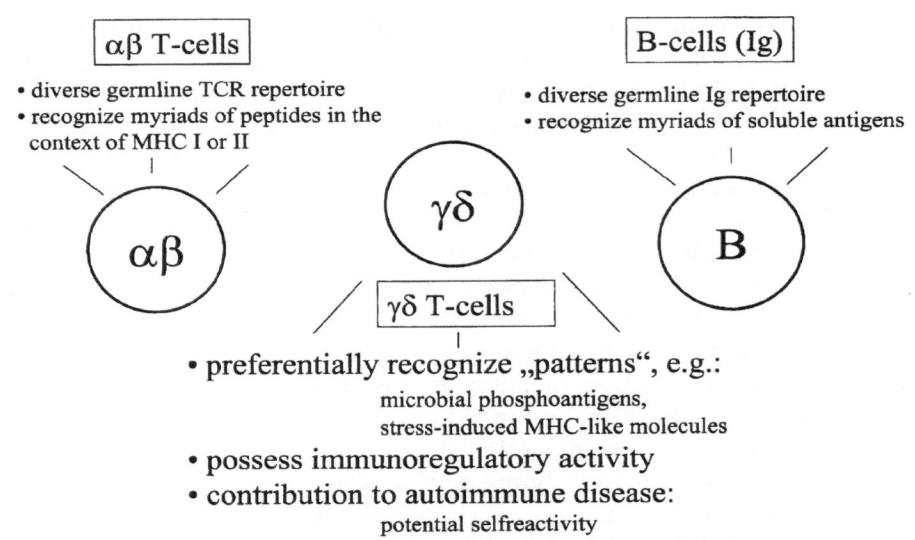

Fig. 2. γδ T cells: a bridge between innate and adaptive immune system? γδ T cells share with αβ T cells and B lymphocytes antigen-specific receptors which, however, they frequently use to recognize "patterns" (e.g., stressed cells, bacterial metabolites) rather than MHC-restricted peptides

this capacity of γδ T cells in more detail for future clinical application, e.g., in the treatment of selected autoimmune diseases.

Acknowledgment. Work from my laboratory received financial support from the Deutsche Forschungsgemeinschaft (Ka 502/6-3, Ka 502/7-2).

References

Allison TJ, Winter CC, Fournié JJ, Bonneville M, Garboczi DN (2001) Structure of a human γδ T-cell antigen receptor. Nature 411: 820–824

Altincicek B, Moll J, Campos N, Foerster G, Beck E, Hoeffler J-F, Grosdemange-Billiard C, Rodríguez-Concepción M, Rohmer M, Boronat A, Eberl M, Jomaa H (2001) Cutting edge: human γδ T cells are activated by intermediates of the 2-C-methyl-D-erythriol 4-phosphate pathway of isoprenoid biosynthesis. J Immunol 166: 3655–3658

Arden B, Clark SP, Kabelitz D, Mak T (1995) Human T-cell receptor variable gene segment families. Immunogenetics 42: 455–500

Belmant C, Espinosa E, Poupot R, Peyrat MA, Guiraud M, Poquet Y, Bonneville M, Fournié JJ (1999) 3-Formyl-1-butyl pyrophosphate: a novel mycobacterial metabolite activating human γδ T cells. J Biol Chem 274: 32079–32084

Boismenu R, Havran WL (1994) Modulation of epithelial cell growth by intestinal γδ T cells. Science 266: 1253–1255

Bonneville M, Ito K, Krecko EG, Itohara S, Kappes D, Ishida I, Kanagawa O, Janeway CA, Murphy DB, Tonegawa S (1989) Recognition of a self major histocompatibility complex TL region product by γδ T cell receptors. Proc Natl Acad Sci USA 86: 5928–5932

Born W, Hall L, Dallas A, Boymel J, Shinnick T, Young D, Brennan P, O'Brien R (1990) Recognition of a peptide antigen by heat shock-reactive γδ T lymphocytes. Science 249: 67–69

Borsellino G, Koul O, Placido R, Tramonti D, Luchetti S, Galgani S, Salvetti M, Gasperini C, Ristori G, Bonetti B, Bach S, Cipriani B, Battistini L (2000) Evidence for a role of γδ T cells in demyelinating diseases as determined by activation states and responses to lipid antigens. J Neuroimmunol 107: 124–129

Bukowski JF, Morita CT, Brenner MB (1999) Human γδ T cells recognize alkylamines derived from microbes, edible plants, and tea: implications for innate immunity. Immunity 11: 57–65

Chien Y-H, Hampl J (2000) Antigen-recognition properties of murine γδ T cells. Springer Semin Immunopathol 22: 239–250

Déchanet J, Merville P, Lim A, Retière C, Pitard V, Lafarge X, Michelson S, Meric C, Hallet M-M, Kourilsky P, Potaux L, Bonneville M, Moreau J-F (1999) Implication of γδ T cells in the human immune response to cytomegalovirus. J Clin Invest 103: 1437–1449

De Libero G (2000) Tissue distribution, antigen specificity and effector functions of γδ T cells in human diseases. Springer Semin Immunopathol 22: 219–238

Deusch K, Lüling F, Rech K, Claasen M, Wagner H, Pfeffer K (1991) A major fraction of human intraepithelial lymphocytes simultaneously expresses the γ/δ T cell receptor, CD8 accessory molecule and preferentially uses the Vδ1 gene segment. Eur J Immunol 21: 1053–1059

Groh V, Steinle A, Bauer S, Spies T (1998) Recognition of stress-induced MHC molecules by intestinal epithelial γδ T cells. Science 279: 1737–1740

Halary F, Peyrat MA, Champagne E, Lopez-Botet M, Moretta A, Moretta L, Viè H, Fournié JJ, Bonneville M (1997) Control of self-reactive cytotoxic T lymphocytes expressing γδ T cell receptors by natural killer inhibitory receptors. Eur J Immunol 27: 2812–2821

Halstensen TS, Scott H, Brandzaeg P (1989) Intraepithelial T cells of the TCR γδ CD8- and Vδ 1/Jδ 1+ phenotypes are increased in celiac disease. Scand J Immunol 30: 665–672

Hanninen A, Harrison LC (2000) γδ T cells as mediators of mucosal tolerance: the autoimmune diabetes model. Immunol Rev 173: 109–119

Harrison LC, Dempsey-Collier M, Kramer DR, Takahashi K (1996) Aerosol insulin induces regulatory CD8 γδ T cells that prevent murine insulin-dependent diabetes. J Exp Med 184: 2167–2174

Havran WL, Chien YH, Allison JP (1991) Recognition of self antigens by skin-derived T cells with invariant γδ antigen receptors. Science 252: 1430–1432

Hayday AC (2000) γδ cells: a right time and a right place for a conserved third way of protection. Annu Rev Immunol 18: 975–1026

Hayday A, Geng L (1997) γδ cells regulate autoimmunity. Curr Opin Immunol 9: 884–889

Hinz T, Wesch D, Friese K, Reckziegel A, Arden B, Kabelitz D (1994) The T cell receptor γδ repertoire in HIV-1 infected individuals. Eur J Immunol 24: 3044–3049

Hinz T, Wesch D, Halary F, Marx S, Choudhary A, Arden B, Janssen O, Bonneville M, Kabelitz D (1997) Identification of the complete expressed human T-cell receptor Vγ repertoire by flow cytometry. Int Immunol 9: 1065–1072

Hohlfeld R, Engel AG, Ii K, Harper MC (1991) Polymyositis mediated by T lymphocytes that express the γ/δ receptor. N Engl J Med 324: 877–881

Kabelitz D, Bender A, Prospero T, Wesselborg S, Janssen O, Pechhold K (1991) The primary response of human γδ+ T cells to Mycobacterium tuberculosis is restricted to Vγ9-bearing cells. J Exp Med 173: 1331–1338

Kabelitz D, Wesch D, Hinz T (1999) γδ T cells, their TCR usage and role in human diseases. Springer Semin Immunopathol 21: 55–75

Kabelitz D, Glatzel A, Wesch D (2000) Antigen recognition by human γδ T lymphocytes. Int Arch Allergy Immunol 122: 1–7

Keystone E, Rittershaus C, Wood N, Snow K, Flatow J, Purvis J (1991) Elevation of a γδ T cell subset in peripheral blood and synovial fluid of patients with rheumatoid arthritis. Clin Exp Immunol 84: 78–82

Komano H, Fujiura Y, Kawaguchi M, Matsumoto M, Hashimoto Y, Obana S, Mombaerts P, Tonegawa S, Yamamoto H, Itohara S, Nanno M, Ishikawa H (1995) Homeostatic regulation of intestinal epithelia by intraepithelial γδ T cells. Proc Natl Acad Sci USA 92: 6147–6151

Morita CT, Mariuzza RA, Brenner MB (2000) Antigen recognition by human γδ T cells: pattern recognition by the adaptive immune system. Springer Semin Immunopathol 22: 191–217

Parker CM, Groh V, Band H, Porcelli SA, Morita G, Fabbi M, Glass D, Strominger JB, Brenner MB (1990) Evidence for extrathymic changes in the T-cell receptor γδ repertoire. J Exp Med 171: 1597

Peng SL, Madaio MP, Hayday AC, Craft J (1996) Propagation and regulation of systemic autoimmunity by γδ T cells. J Immunol 157: 5689–5698

Pluschke G, Rügge D, Hohlfeld R, Engel AG (1992) Autoaggressive myocytotoxic T lymphocytes expressing an unusual γ/δ T cell receptor. J Exp Med 176: 1785–1789

Porcelli SA, Brenner MB, Band H (1991) Biology of the human γδ T-cell receptor. Immunol Rev 120: 137–183

Rajagopalan S, Zordan T, Tsokos GC, Datta SK (1990) Pathogenic anti-DNA autoantibody-inducing T helper cell lines from patients with acute lupus nephritis: isolation of CD4⁻8⁻ T helper cell lines that express the γδ T-cell antigen receptor. Proc Natl Acad Sci USA 87: 7020–7024

Rajan AJ, Klein JDS, Brosnan CF (1998) The effect of γδ T cell depletion on cytokine gene expression in experimental allergic encephalomyelitis. J Immunol 160: 5955–5962

Schild H, Mavaddat N, Litzenberger C, Ehrlich EW, Davis MM, Bluestone JB, Matis L, Draper RK, Chien Y-H (1994) The nature of major histocompatibilty complex recognition by γδ T-cells. Cell 76: 29–37

Sciammas R, Johnson RM, Sperling AI, Brady W, Linsley PS, Spear PG, Fitch FW, Bluestone JA (1994) Unique antigen recognition by a herpesvirus-specific TCR-γδ cells. J Immunol 152: 5392–5397

Selmaj K, Brosnan CF, Raine CS (1991) Colocalization of lymphocytes bearing γδ T cell receptor and heat shock protein hsp65⁺ oligodendrocytes in multiple sclerosis. Proc Natl Acad Sci USA 88: 6452–6456

Shevach EM (2000) Regulatory cells in autoimmunity. Annu Rev Immunol 18: 423–449

Spada FM, Grant EP, Peters PJ, Sugita M, Melián A, Lesile DS, Lee HK, van Donselar E, Hanson DA, Krensky AM, Majdic O, Porcelli SA, Morita CT, Brenner MB (2000) Self recognition of CD1 by γδ T cells: implications for innate immunity. J Exp Med 191: 937–948

Wesch D, Hinz T, Kabelitz D (1998) Analysis of the T cell receptor Vγ repertoire in healthy donors and HIV-1 infected individuals. Int Immunol 10: 1067–1075

Weintraub BC, Jackson MR, Hedrick SM (1994) Gamma delta T cells can recognize nonclassical MHC in the absence of conventional antigenic peptides. J Immunol 153: 3051–3058

Wildner G, Hünig T, Thurau SR (1996) Orally induced, peptide-specific γ/δ TCR⁺ cells suppress experimental autoimmune uveitis. Eur J Immunol 26: 2140–2148

Yin Z, Craft J (2000) γδ T cells in autoimmunity. Springer Semin Immunopathol 22: 311–320

Zeine R, Pon R, Ladiwala U, Antel JP, Filion LG, Freedman MS (1998) Mechanism of γδ T cell-induced human oligodendrocyte cytotoxicity: relevance to multiple sclerosis. J Neuroimmunol 87: 49–61

Treatment of autoimmune diseases by targeted DNA vaccines encoding proinflammatory mediators

Nathan Karin*

Department of Immunology, Rappaport Faculty of Medicine and Rappaport Institute
for Medical Sciences, Technion Israel Institute of Technology, Haifa, Israel

Therapeutic concepts of gene therapy and DNA vaccination for immunological disorders

Conceptually, gene therapy has been used as an efficient methodology to circumvent genetic deficiency by transfection of cDNA encoding the appropriate functional gene product. It is therefore conceivable that best candidates for this way of therapy would be genetic diseases associated with a single-gene mutation, such as X-linked agammaglobulinemia or cystic fibrosis. Paradoxically, it appears that gene therapy needs to confront similar levels of technological challenges when encountering genetic disorders, such as X-linked agammaglobulinemia or cystic fibrosis, to those required for a successful intervention in multifactorial diseases. Yet, while genetic disorders that evolve a mutation in a single gene are rare, multifactorial diseases are a major cause of illness and death in the developed countries. This has motivated scientists to explore gene therapy strategies in multifactorial disorders. The current review discusses the use of a modification of gene therapy named DNA vaccination to suggest novel ways for interfering in the regulation of the inflammatory process in T-cell-mediated autoimmune diseases, such as multiple sclerosis (MS), rheumatoid arthritis (RA), and others.

One approach for applying gene therapy in T-cell-mediated autoimmunity evolves in vitro transfection of antigen-specific autoimmune T cells with a regulatory gene of interest, such as IL-4 (interleukin-4) or IL-10 (Shaw et al. 1997, Mathisen and Tuohy 1998). Upon injecting the manipulated T cells into the circulation the cells are expected to home to the target autoimmune organ and propagate

* Author's address: Department of Immunology, Rappaport Faculty of Medicine, Technion Israel Institute of Technology, Haifa 32000, Israel.

the response to the specific autoimmune determinate (Shaw et al. 1997, Mathisen and Tuohy 1998). While so doing they produce and secrete the desired regulatory gene product at this site and restrain the relevant autoimmune disease (Shaw et al. 1997, Mathisen and Tuohy 1998). My group has utilized another modification of gene therapy, by which the immune system could be "re-educated" to restrain its harmful activities. In contrast to "classical" gene therapy, our strategy "only" uses plasmid DNA vaccines encoding gene products of interest to elicit protective immunity against their gene products.

Basic experimental models

Experimental autoimmune encephalomyelitis (EAE) is a paralytic autoimmune disease of the central nervous system that serves as an animal model for MS. In both diseases, circulating leukocytes enter the blood brain to interact with their target antigens, resulting in impaired nerve conduction and paralysis. The disease could be induced in various susceptible strains of animals, one of which is the Lewis strain of rats. Upon a single immunization with myelin basic protein (MBP) emulsified in an appropriate adjuvant these rats develop active EAE (Ben-Nun et al. 1981a). MBP-specific CD4$^+$ T cell clones and lines selected from EAE rats are capable of transferring the disease to naive recipients (Ben-Nun et al. 1981a). When being attenuated to become nonencephalitogenic, or if administered at a subpathogenic dose, these cells can endow recipients a high state of resistance against any further attempt to induce the disease (Ben-Nun et al. 1981b, Beraud et al. 1989, Lider et al. 1989). The suggested mechanism included elicitation of self-specific anti-idiotypic response, which includes CD4$^+$ (Lider et al. 1989) and CD8$^+$ (Sun et al. 1988a, b) regulatory T cells. These studies suggest that some cells of the specific arm of the immune system not only do not participate in the induction of antigen-specific effector function but also regulate the harmful function of autoimmune effector T cells. As discussed below, my group has recently defined another mechanism by which immune cells mount an immune response against self-antigens (proinflammatory cytokines and chemokines) to restrain the harmful activity of autoimmune T cells. Two other models are the relapsing-remitting disease in the SJL mice and the semichronic disease in the C57BL6 mice. These experimentally induced diseases represent relapsing-remitting and chronic progressive MS and are of a major interest in our laboratory. At the moment we are extending basic findings that are described below to these models.

As a key comparative model we are using adjuvant-induced arthritis (AA) in the same strain of rats. Depending on the mode of immunization, a single administration of complete Freund adjuvant (CFA) may result in the development of a local inflammatory process or chronic poly adjuvant-induced arthritis (Pearson 1956). Under our working condition the disease is chronic and histologically and clinically well resembles human RA (Youssef et al. 2000). In both diseases, proinflammatory cytokines and chemokines are believed to play a pivotal role in the attraction of leukocytes to the site of inflammation and in the initiation and progression of the inflammatory process.

Role of cytokines and chemokines in development and progression of T-cell-mediated autoimmunity

The role of cytokines and chemokines in the regulation of T-cell-mediated auto-immunity has been extensively studied. On the basis of their cytokine profile CD4[+] T-cells can be divided into Th1 cells, which produce large amounts of gamma interferon (IFN-γ) and tumor necrosis factor alpha (TNF-α) and, to a much lesser extent, IL-4 and IL-10, and Th2 cells, which produce IL-4, IL-10, and IL-13 and, to a much lesser extent, IFN-γ and TNF-α (Mosmann and Coffman 1989; Mosmann and Moore 1991; Swain et al. 1990; Fiorentino et al. 1991; Seder et al. 1992, 1993; O'Garra and Murphy 1994; Abbas et al. 1996; Lederer et al. 1996; Huang et al. 1997). More recently defined subsets are the Th3 cells, which produce significant amounts of transforming growth factor beta (TGF-β) and have been associated with oral tolerance (Fukaura et al. 1996), and the high IL-10- and low IL-4-producing regulatory T cells that have been implicated with colitis (Groux et al. 1997). Th1 cells selected in response to various auto-antigens transfer T-cell-mediated autoimmune diseases, whereas IL-4-secreting Th2 cells, selected in response to these same antigens, either inhibit or exert no profound effect on the inflammatory process (Ando et al. 1989, Rapoport et al. 1993, Saoudi et al. 1993, Sedes et al. 1993, Trinchieri et al. 1993, Cash et al. 1994, Racke et al. 1994, Rott et al. 1994, Healey et al. 1995, Katz et al. 1995, Khoruts et al. 1995, Kuchroo et al. 1995, Liblau et al. 1995, Leonard et al. 1995). High levels of IFN-γ and low levels of IL-4 positively select for Th1 cells, whereas low levels of IFN-γ together with high levels of IL-4 mediate Th2 selection (Swain et al. 1990; Seder et al. 1992, 1993; O'Garra and Murphy 1994; Abbas et al. 1996; Lederer et al. 1996). In a recent study Wildbaum et al. (1998) isolated mRNA encoding rat IFN-γ-inducing factor (IGIF, IL-18) from the EAE brain, generated neutralizing antibodies against its gene product, and used them to explore the role of IGIF in T cell deviation and function. These antibodies significantly reduced the production of IFN-γ by primed T cells proliferating in response to their target MBP epitope and by concanavalin A-activated T cells from naive donors. When administered to rats during the development of either active or transferred EAE, these antibodies significantly blocked the development of disease. T cells from protected rats were cultured with the encephalitogenic MBP epitope and evaluated for production of IL-4 and IFN-γ. These cells, which proliferated, exhibited a profound increase in IL-4 production, accompanied by a significant decrease in IFN-γ and TNF-α production (Wildbaum et al. 1998). This study demonstrated, again, that by simple means one may interfere in a natural mechanism by which self-tolerance is maintained by the peripheral immune system to keep autoreactive lymphocytes under control.

Likewise, anti-chemokine therapy by either antibodies or antagonists was found to be effective in blocking the development or progression of T-cell-mediated autoimmune diseases. Chemokines are chemoattractants that mediate leukocyte attraction and recruitment. As such, they are likely to be key mediators in the massive recruitment of leukocytes at the site of inflammation during the course of T-cell-mediated inflammatory conditions, including autoimmune disorders. On the basis of the positions of the first two cysteines, the chemokines can be divided into four highly conserved but distinct supergene families, C-C, C-X-C, C, and C-X3-C (Bazan et al. 1997, Pan et al. 1997, Rollins 1997, Sallusto et al. 1998, Ward et al. 1998). The C-C family is primarily involved in the activation of endothelium and chemoattraction of T cells and monocytes to the site of inflammation. This has motivated several investigators, including us, to explore anti C-C chemokine immunity as a potential way of suppressing EAE and other T-cell-mediated auto-immune diseases. About six years ago Karpus et al. (1995) blocked EAE in mice by immunizing them with rabbit anti-mouse polyclonal antibody against macro-phage inflammatory protein-1α (MIP-1α). Thereafter Gong et al. (1997) used an antagonist of monocyte chemoattractant protein 1 (MCP-1) to inhibit arthritis in the MRL-*lpr* mouse model. Later Barnes et al. (1998) used anti-human RANTES to ameliorate adjuvant-induced arthritis in the Lewis rat. As with proinflammatory cytokines, effective therapy requires a continuing administration of antibodies or antichemokine antagonists.

As an alternative approach to treat T-cell-mediated autoimmune diseases one may use antibodies to key adhesion molecules that mediate leukocyte migration to their target organ. Ten years ago we (Yednock et al. 1992) have defined the alpha-4 beta 1 integrin (VLA-4) as the key adhesion molecule that mediates T cells and monocyte trans-migration to the target autoimmune site in EAE and demonstrated that VLA-4-specific antibodies can inhibit the development and progression of disease. The underlying mechanism includes blockade of the secondary influx of leukocytes that is required for the development and progression of disease (Karin et al. 1993). Once again, this way of therapy is not disease- or organ-specific and is dependent on a continuing exposure to these antibodies.

In an attempt to develop a highly specific therapeutic strategy we have explored the competence of dominant epitopes of MBP, or even soluble altered analogs of these epitopes, to inhibit an ongoing disease (Karin et al. 1994, 1998; Brocke et al. 1996). In a recent study we (Karin et al. 1998) have demonstrated that an engage-ment of the antigenic determinant to one MHC anchor and to one TCR binding site of an MBP determinant could be sufficient for the generation antigen-specific T cell tolerance, whereas 5 to 7 simultaneous engagements of an MBP determinant to MHC and TCR are required for mounting an encephalitogenic response in self-reactive T cells. Perhaps during the evolution of self–non-self recognition the immune system has been evolved to induce self-specific unresponsiveness more readily than self-specific proinflammatory response. The major advantage of using such a nonpathogenic altered antigen analog for therapy resides in its specificity. Yet as with previous means of therapy discussed above it requires a continuing administration, which is impractical for the treatment of long-lasting chronic diseases.

Targeted DNA vaccines, an alternative way for treating long-lasting autoimmune diseases

An ideal way to treat a T-cell-mediated autoimmune condition is by redirecting the immune system to use the tools with which it generates autoimmunity to generate protective immunity. In several recent studies we have recorded the development of an apparent autoimmune response (anti-self-antibody titer) to proinflammatory mediators such as TNF-α and several chemokines in animals with developing AA or EAE. We are now extending these studies to MS and RA patients. Our basic theory is that in order to maintain a wide repertoire of antigen-specific T and B cells, many autoreactive lymphocytes should escape central selection. This potentially increases the chance of developing destructive autoimmunity. One way by which evolution have been dealing with this complicated issue is by directing some of these autoreactive T cells that escape central selection to become regulatory cells that produce neutralizing antibodies to proinflammatory mediators of the immune system, such as TNF-α and proinflammatory chemokines (Youssef et al. 1998, 1999; Wildbaum and Karin 1999). That is, antichemokine and -cytokine antigen-specific B cells produce antibodies in a T-cell-dependent manner, and that this response is regulated by the development and progression of an autoimmune condition and not by a local inflammatory process (Youssef et al. 1998, 1999; Wildbaum and Karin 1999). As this response is not sufficient to prevent the development and progression of an autoimmune condition, we have looked for ways by which this response could be amplified in accordance to the development and progression of the autoimmune condition. For this purpose we have selected a modification of gene therapy named naked DNA vaccination. A major current use of this technology is for the increase of cell-mediated antigen-specific immune response against infectious agents such as tuberculosis, HIV, and allergens such as mite proteins (Raz et al. 1993, 1999; Sato et al. 1996; Tascon et al. 1996; Boyer et al. 1997; Kim et al. 1997a, b). The interesting work of Waisman et al. (1996) paved the way for applying this powerful technology to elicit protective immunity to experimental autoimmune diseases. In their study, Waisman et al. (1996) inhibited EAE by immunizing mice with cDNA encoding the T cell receptor V genes. In our studies we (Wildbaum and Karin 1999, Youssef et al. 1998) tried to use naked DNA vaccination to breakdown the tolerance to proinflammatory mediators of the autoimmune process, thus generating immunological memory against these proinflammatory factors. Thus each gene of interest was cloned into a mammalian vector with a strong viral promoter (cytomegalovirus) and a repeated immunostimulatory sequence (ISS) (Raz et al. 1996, Sato et al. 1996). We have demonstrated that upon repeated administrations of each vaccine the tolerance to its gene product was broken and immunological memory was established (Wildbaum and Karin 1999, Youssef et al. 1998). The mechanistic basis by which ISS acts as a DNA adjuvant has recently been explored. Two independent, yet complementary, studies have shown that the ISS activate a signaling cascade, probably via Toll receptor 9 leading to the activation of antigen-presenting cells of the innate immune system (i.e., dendritic cells and macrophages) that present the product of the inserted gene and thus allow the breakdown of tolerance to self (Chu et al. 2000, Hemmi et al. 2000, Modlin 2000).

At first we have used this strategy to generate protective immunity. That is, rats were immunized with MBP-CFA to induce active EAE two months after the last administration of each vaccine. At this time the self-specific antibody titer to each gene product regressed back to background levels. Interestingly, immunization with MBP-CFA to induce active EAE, and not with the CFA alone, to elicit a local inflammatory process, elicited the rapid production of self-specific antibodies to the product of each given vaccine (Wildbaum and Karin 1999, Youssef et al. 1998). Thus, rats that were previously subjected to naked DNA vaccines encoding MIP-1α, MCP-1, or TNF-α were EAE resistant and at that time exhibited a marked antibody titer against the gene product of each vaccine. Each titer accelerated in accordance with the progression of disease in control EAE rats and regressed back to background levels upon recovery. MCP-1-, MIP-1α- and TNF-α-specific antibodies generated in EAE-resistant rats were neutralizing in vitro and could transfer EAE resistance in adoptive transfer experiments (Wildbaum and Karin 1999, Youssef et al. 1998). Thus by applying proinflammatory cytokine- and chemokine-based naked DNA vaccination one may reeducate the immune system to use self-specific immunity to restrain its own harmful activities (Wildbaum and Karin 1999, Youssef et al. 1998). We have also used this interesting strategy to breakdown the tolerance to FAS ligand (FasL) and used the anti-FasL autoantibodies to explore the distinct functions of FasL in the regulation of T-cell-mediated autoimmunity (Wildbaum et al. 2000a). In this particular study we have shown that an early administration of such antibodies prevents apoptosis of central nervous system residual cells that appears to be important for the progression of the autoimmune cascade. Later administration of these antibodies exhibits an opposing effect by inhibiting the entry of autoimmune T cells to programmed cell death, thus prolonging the length and severity of disease (Wildbaum et al. 2000a).

In another two recent studies we have explored the ability of targeted DNA vaccines encoding TNF-α or various chemokines to treat an ongoing form of long-lasting AA. It appears that administration of these vaccines, not only at the early stage but also during a full-blown disease, led recipients to a fast long-lasting remission that was not dependent on a continued exposure to the vaccine (Youssef et al. 2000, Wildbaum et al. 2000b). From this perspective the treatment holds an apparent advantage over soluble receptor and humanized antibody therapy. Surprisingly, the production of neutralizing antibodies to the gene product of these vaccines accelerated within 2–3 days after treatment, as if DNA vaccines accelerate a pre-existing network (Wildbaum et al. 2000b).

The biological significance of the association between the elevated levels of proinflammatory mediators mRNA at a privileged autoimmune site (central nervous system) and the enhancement in anti-self response against proinflammatory cytokines and chemokines is apparent. After all, an ideal immune system would be selected in evolution to centralize its destructive competence against invading microbes rather than against the self-tissues it was designed to protect (Janeway 1992, Matzinger 1994, Steinmann 1995). The underlying mechanism by which the immune system distinguishes a gene product transcribed at a privileged autoimmune site from the same gene product transcribed at a local site of inflammation is however still elusive. A partial explanation for these intriguing observations was previously suggested by Goodnow and his colleagues (Cyster et al. 1994). This group brought compelling evidence to suggest that peripheral clonal exclusion of self-reactive B cells occurs in germinal centers of lymph nodes that drain tissues lacking immune surveillance (i.e., immune privileged areas), where competition for follicular niches does not exclude self-reactive cells from the recirculating B cell repertoire (Cyster et al. 1994). This may suggest that the expression and production of proinflammatory cytokines and chemokines will lead to the exclusion of self-specific B cells, capable of generating an immune response to these self-gene products, unless they are transcribed and produced at an autoimmune site, such as the central nervous system (Cyster et al. 1994). Proinflammatory chemokine- and cytokine-based DNA vaccination probably amplifies this process of tolerance breakdown. Alternatively, it could be that memory B cells enter the autoimmune site where these proinflammatory mediators are being largely produced, and as long as the inflammatory autoimmune condition continues, the production of anti-inflammatory immunity proceeds. From the basic-science perspective, the above observations may provide a new perspective for understanding the role of T cell and B cell selection in the induction and maintenance of tolerance to self. In the process of negative selection, self-reactive T cells die when they encounter self-antigen in the thymus (Kappler et al. 1987, Ramsdell and Fowlkes 1990). Similarly, self-specific pre-B cells either die or undergo receptor editing in the bone marrow (Melamed et al. 1998). It is believed that those cells escaping central tolerance are subjected to various mechanisms acting outside the thymus or the bone marrow to keep them under control. This type of control has been termed peripheral tolerance. T cell anergy (Friedman and Weiner 1994), active suppression (Khoury et al. 1992, Saoudi et al. 1993, Friedman et al. 1994, Chen et al. 1994), T cell deletion (Critchfield et al. 1994, Critchfield and Lenardo 1995), and generation of anti-idiotypic immunity (Lider et al. 1988) have been described as key mechanisms that contribute to the maintenance of peripheral tolerance. The current study suggests for the first time that self-specific T and B cells, capable of mounting self-specific immunity against proinflammatory mediators, escape central tolerance to provide the immune system a powerful tool with which it keeps its dangerous anti-self activity under control and thus maintains tolerance to self in the periphery. Moreover, as microbes and self-components are constructed from similar "building blocks" and as central selection manifests its own limitations, anti-self immunity cannot be avoided but rather has to be restrained by peripheral mechanisms. Moreover, it could well be that a substantial increase in the competence of the immune system to effectively limit its T and B cell repertoire would result in a constrained ability to effectively confront infectious diseases. The case of natural immunity to TNF-α, evoked during the course of a T-cell-mediated autoimmune disease, demonstrates how the immune system has evolved to benefit from its own limited competence to effectively select against self-reactivity.

From a clinical perspective, the advantage of interfering in the autoimmune process by cytokine and chemokine DNA vaccines is apparent. A major disadvantage in treating chronic diseases with xenogenic neutralizing antibodies lies in their immunogenicity. This has motivated investigators to develop chimeric humanized antibodies (reviewed in Riethmüller et al. 1992) and monoclonal antibodies engineered with human immunoglobulin heavy and light chain yeast artificial chromosome (Green et al. 1994). However, following repeated immunization, these engineered antibodies do trigger an apparently allotypic response. The therapeutic strategy suggested by our studies is of advantage over the above methods since it results in the generation of immunity to autologous antigen only during the course of disease at the time when the mRNA level encoding the proinflammatory cytokine is profoundly elicited at the site of inflammation. Yet another major disadvantage of applying antichemokine and -cytokine immunotherapy in T-cell-mediated autoimmunity is that the treatment is not disease specific and may lead to suppression or alteration of other immunological functions. Ultimately, an ideal DNA vaccine would exert a maximal effect on the clinical manifestation of an autoimmune condition with a minimal effect on other immunological functions. We believe that the next breakthrough in the development of genetic vaccines for T-cell-mediated autoimmunity would depend on defining disease-specific chemokine- and cytokine-encoding DNA vaccines. This goal is still dependent on the future characterization of organ-specific and disease-specific proinflammatory factors.

References

Abbas AK, Murphy KM, Sher A (1996) Functional diversity of helper T lymphocytes. Nature 383: 787–793

Ando DG, Clayton J, Kono D, Urban JL, Sercarz EE (1989) Encephalitogenic T cells in the B10.PL model of experimental allergic encephalomyelitis (EAE) are of the Th-1 lymphokine subtype. Cell Immunol 124: 132–143

Barnes DA, Tse J, Kaufhold M, Owen M, Hesselgesser J, Strieter R, et al (1998) Polyclonal antibody directed against human RANTES ameliorates disease in the Lewis rat adjuvant-induced arthritis model. J Clin Invest 101: 2910–2919

Bazan JF, Bacon KB, Hardiman G, Wang W, Soo K, Rossi D, et al (1997) A new class of membrane-bound chemokine with a CX3C motif. Nature 385: 640–644

Ben-Nun A, Wekerle H, Cohen IR (1981a) The rapid isolation of clonable antigen-specific T lymphocyte lines capable of mediating autoimmune encephalomyelitis. Eur J Immunol 11: 195–199

Ben-Nun A, Wekerle H, Cohen IR (1981b) Vaccination against autoimmune encephalomyelitis with T-lymphocyte line cells reactive against myelin basic protein. Nature 292: 60–61

Beraud E, Lider O, Baharav E, Reshef T, Cohen IR (1989) Vaccination against experimental autoimmune encephalomyelitis using a subencephalitogenic dose of autoimmune effector cells 1: characteristics of vaccination. J Autoimmun 2: 75–86

Boyer JD, Ugen KE, Wang B, Agadjanyan M, Gilbert L, Bagarazzi ML, et al (1997) Protection of chimpanzees from high-dose heterologous HIV-1 challenge by DNA vaccination. Nat Med 3: 526–532

Brocke S, Gijbels K, Allegretta M, Ferber I, Piercy C, Blankenstein T, et al (1996) Treatment of experimental encephalomyelitis with a peptide analogue of myelin basic protein. Nature 379: 343–346

Cash E, Minty A, Ferrara P, Caput D, Fradelizi D, Rott O (1994) Macrophage-inactivating IL-13 suppresses experimental autoimmune encephalomyelitis in rats. J Immunol 153: 4258–4267

Chen Y, Kuchroo VK, Inobe J, Hafler D, Weiner HL (1994) Regulatory T-cell clones induced by oral tolerance: suppression of autoimmune encephalomyelitis. Science 265: 1237–1240

Chu W, Gong X, Li Z, Takabayash K, Ouyang H, Chen Y, et al (2000) DNA-PKcs is required for activation of innate immunity by immunostimulatory DNA. Cell 103: 909–918

Critchfield JM, Lenardo MJ (1995) Antigen-induced programmed T cell death as a new approach to immune therapy. Clin Immunol Immunopathol 75: 13–19

Critchfield JM, Racke MK, Zuniga PJ, Cannella B, Raine CS, Goverman J, et al (1994) T cell deletion in high antigen dose therapy of autoimmune encephalomyelitis. Science 263: 1139–1143

Cyster JG, Hartley SB, Goodnow CC (1994) Competition for follicular niches excludes self-reactive cells from the recirculating B-cell repertoire. Nature 371: 389–395

Fiorentino DF, Zlotnik A, Vieira P, Mosmann TR, Howard M, Moore KW, et al (1991) IL-10 acts on the antigen presenting cell to inhibit cytokine production by Th1 cells. J Immunol 146: 3444–3451

Friedman A, Weiner HL (1994) Induction of anergy or active suppression following oral tolerance is determined by antigen dosage. Proc Natl Acad Sci USA 91: 6688–6692

Fukaura H, Kent SC, Pietrusewicz MJ, Khoury SJ, Weiner HL, Hafler DA (1996) Induction of circulating myelin basic protein and proteolipid protein-specific transforming growth factor-beta1-secreting Th3 T cells by oral administration of myelin in multiple sclerosis patients. J Clin Invest 98: 70–77

Gong JH, Ratkay LG, Waterfield JD, Clark-Lewis I (1997) An antagonist of monocyte chemoattractant protein 1 (MCP-1) inhibits arthritis in the MRL-1pr mouse model. J Exp Med 186: 131–137

Green LL, Hardy MC, Maynard-Currie CE, Tsuda H, Louie DM, Mendez MJ, et al (1994) Antigen-specific human monoclonal antibodies from mice engineered with human Ig heavy and light chain YACs. Nat Genet 7: 13–21

Groux H, O'Garra A, Bigler M, Rouleau M, Antonenko S, de Vries JE, et al (1997) A CD4+ T-cell subset inhibits antigen-specific T-cell responses and prevents colitis. Nature 389: 737–742

Healey D, Ozegbe P, Arden S, Chandler P, Hutton J, Cooke A (1995) In vivo activity and in vitro specificity of CD4+ Th1 and Th2 cells derived from the spleens of diabetic NOD mice. J Clin Invest 95: 2979–2985

Hemmi H, Takeuchi O, Kawai T, Kaisho T, Sato S, Sanjo H, et al (2000) A Toll-like receptor recognizes bacterial DNA. Nature 408: 740–745

Huang H, Hu-Li J, Chen H, Ben-Sasson SZ, Paul WE (1997) IL-4 and IL-13 production in differentiated T helper type 2 cells is not IL-4 dependent. J Immunol 159: 3731–3738

Janeway CA Jr (1992) The immune system evolved to discriminate infectious nonself from noninfectious self. Immunol Today 13: 11–16

Kappler J, Roehm N, Marrack P (1987) T cell tolerance by clonal elemination in the thymus. Cell 49: 273–280

Karin N, Szafer F, Mitchell D, Gold DP, Steinman L (1993) Selective and nonselective stages in homing of T lymphocytes to the central nervous system during experimental allergic encephalomyelitis. J Immunol 150: 4116–4124

Karin N, Mitchell JD, Brocke S, Ling N, Steinman L (1994) Reversal of experimental autoimmune encephalomyelitis by as soluble peptide variant of a myelin basic protein epitope: T cell receptor antagonism and reduction of IFN-g and TNF-a production. J Exp Med 180: 2227–2237

Karin N, Binah O, Grabie N, Mitchel DJ, Felzen B, Solomon MD, et al (1998) Short peptide based tolerogens without antigenic activity reverse autoimmunity. J Immunol 160: 5188–5149

Karpus WJ, Lukacs NW, McRae BL, Strieter RM, Kunkel SL, Miller SD (1995) An important role for the chemokine macrophage inflammatory protein-1 alpha in the pathogenesis of the T cell-mediated autoimmune disease, experimental autoimmune encephalomyelitis. J Immunol 155: 5003–5010

Katz JD, Benoist C, Mathis D (1995) T helper subsets in insulin dependent diabetes. Science 268: 1185–1188

Khoruts A, Miller SD, Jenkins MK (1995) Neuroantigen-specific Th2 cells are inefficient suppressors of experimental autoimmune encephalomyelitis induced by effector Th1 cells. J Immunol 155: 5011–5017

Khoury SJ, Hancock WW, Weiner HL (1992) Oral tolerance to myelin basic protein and natural recovery from experimental autoimmune encephalomyelitis are associated with downregulation of inflammatory cytokines and differential upregulation of transforming growth factor beta, interleukin 4, and prostaglandin E expression in the brain. J Exp Med 176: 1355–1364

Kim JJ, Ayyavoo V, Bagarazzi ML, Chattergoon MA, Dang K, Wang B, et al (1997a) In vivo engineering of a cellular immune response by coadministration of IL-12 expression vector with a DNA immunogen. J Immunol 158: 816–826

Kim JJ, Bagarazzi ML, Trivedi N, Hu Y, Kazahaya K, Wilson DM, et al (1997b) Engineering of in vivo immune responses to DNA immunization via codelivery of costimulatory molecule genes. Nat Biotechnol 15: 641–646

Kuchroo VK, Das MP, Brown JA, Ranger AM, Zamvil SS, Sobel RA, et al (1995) B7-1 and B7-2 costimulatory molecules activate differentially the Th1/Th2 developmental pathways: application to autoimmune disease therapy. Cell 80: 707–718

Lederer JA, Perez VL, DesRoches L, Kim SM, Abbas AK, Lichtman AH (1996) Cytokine transcriptional events during helper T cell subset differentiation. J Exp Med 184: 397–406

Leonard JP, Waldburger KE, Goldman SJ (1995) Prevention of experimental autoimmune encephalomyelitis by antibodies against interleukin 12. J Exp Med 181: 381–386

Liblau RS, Singer SM, McDevitt HO (1995) Th1 and Th2 CD4+ T-cells in the pathogenesis of organ-specific autoimmune diseases. Immunol Today 16: 34–38

Lider O, Reshef T, Beraud E, Ben-Nun A, Cohen IR (1988) Anti-idiotypic network induced by T cell vaccination against experimental autoimmune encephalomylitis. Science 239: 181–183

Lider O, Beraud E, Reshef T, Friedman A, Cohen IR (1989) Vaccination against experimental autoimmune encephalomyelitis using a subencephalitogenic dose of autoimmune effector T cells 2: induction of a protective anti-idiotypic response. J Autoimmun 2: 87–99

Mathisen PM, Tuohy VK (1998) Gene therapy in treatment of autoimmune diseases. Immunol Today 19: 193–195

Matzinger P (1994) Tolerance, danger, and the extended family. Annu Rev Immunol 12: 991–1045

Melamed D, Benschop RJ, Cambier JC, Nemazee D (1998) Developmental regulation of B lymphocyte immune tolerance compartmentalizes clonal selection from receptor selection. Cell 92: 173–182

Modlin RL (2000) A Toll for DNA vaccine. Nature 408: 659–660

Mosmann TR, Coffman RL (1989) Th1 and Th2 cells: different patterns of lymphokine secretion lead to different functional properties. Annu Rev Immunol 9: 145–173

Mosmann T, Moore K (1991) The role of IL-10 in the crossregulation of Th1 and Th2 responses. Immunol Today 12: A49–A53

O'Garra A, Murphy K (1994) Role of cytokines in determining T-lymphocyte function. Curr Opin Immunol 6: 458–466

Pan Y, Lloyd C, Zhou H, Dolich S, Deeds J, Gonzalo JA, et al (1997) Neurotactin, a membrane-anchored chemokine upregulated in brain inflammation. Nature 387: 611–617

Pearson CM (1956) Development of arthritis, periarthritis and periostitis in rats given adjuvants. Proc Soc Exp Biol Med 91: 95–101

Racke MK, Bonomo A, Scott DE, Cannella B, Levine A, Raine CS, et al (1994) Cytokine-induced immune deviation as a therapy for inflammatory autoimmune disease. J Exp Med 180: 1961–1966

Ramsdell F, Fowlkes BJ (1990) Clonal deletion versus clonal anergy: the role of the thymus in inducing self tolerance. Science 248: 1342–1348

Rapoport MJ, Jaramillo A, Zipris D, Lazarus A, Serreze DV, Leiter EH, et al (1993) Interleukin-4 reverses T cell proliferative unresponsiveness and prevents the onset of diabetes in nonobese diabetic mice. J Exp Med 178: 87–99

Raz E, Watanabe A, Baird SM, Eisenberg RA, Parr TB, Lotz M, et al (1993) Systemic immunological effects of cytokine genes injected into skeletal muscle. Proc Natl Acad Sci USA 90: 4523–4527

Raz E, Tighe H, Sato Y, Corr M, Dudler JA, Roman M, et al (1996) Preferential induction of a Th1 immune response and inhibition of specific IgE antibody formation by plasmid DNA immunization. Proc Natl Acad Sci USA 93: 5141–5145

Riethmuller G, Rieber EP, Kiefersauer S, Prinz J, van der Lubbe P, Meiser B, et al (1992) From antilymphocyte serum to therapeutic monoclonal antibodies: first experiences with a chimeric CD4 antibody in the treatment of autoimmune disease. Immunol Rev 129: 81–104

Rollins BJ (1997) Chemokines. Blood 90: 909–928

Rott O, Fleischer B, Cash E (1994) Interleukin-10 prevents experimental allergic encephalomyelitis in rats. Eur J Immunol 24: 1434–1440

Sallusto F, Lanzavecchia A, Mackay CR (1998) Chemokines and chemokine receptors in T-cell priming and Th1/Th2- mediated responses. Immunol Today 19: 568–574

Saoudi A, Kuhn J, Huygen K, de Kozak Y, Velu T, Goldman M, et al (1993) TH2 activated cells prevent experimental autoimmune uveoretinitis, a TH1-dependent autoimmune disease. Eur J Immunol 23: 3096–3103

Sato Y, Roman M, Tighe H, Lee D, Corr M, Nguyen M, et al (1996) Immunostimulatory DNA sequences necessary for effective intradermal gene immunization. Science 273: 352–354

Seder RA, Paul WE, Davis MM, Fazekas de St. Groth B (1992) The presence of interleukin-4 during in vitro priming determines the cytokine-producing potential of CD4$^+$ T cells from T cell receptor transgenic mice. J Exp Med 176: 1091–1098

Seder RA, Gazzinelli R, Sher A, Paul WE (1993) IL-12 acts directly on CD4$^+$ T cells to enhance priming for IFN-γ production and diminishes IL-4 inhibition of such priming. Proc Natl Acad Sci USA 90: 10188–10192

Shaw MK, Lorens JB, Dhawan A, DalCanto R, Tse HY, Tran AB, et al (1997) Local delivery of interleukin 4 by retrovirus-transduced T lymphocytes ameliorates experimental autoimmune encephalomyelitis. J Exp Med 185: 1711–1714

Steinman L (1995) Escape from "horror autotoxicus": pathogenesis and treatment of autoimmune disease. Cell 80: 7–10

Sun D, Ben-Nun A, Wekerle H (1988a) Regulatory circuits in autoimmunity: recruitment of counter-regulatory CD8[+] T cells by encephalitogenic CD4[+] T line cells. Eur J Immunol 18: 1993–1999

Sun D, Qin Y, Chluba J, Epplen JT, Wekerle H (1988b) Suppression of experimentally induced auto-immune encephalomyelitis by cytolytic T-T cell interactions. Nature 332: 843–845

Swain SL, Weinberg AD, English M, Huston G (1990) IL-4 directs the development of Th2-like helper effectors. J Immunol 145: 3796–3806

Tascon RE, Colston MJ, Ragno S, Stavropoulos E, Gregory D, Lowrie DB (1996) Vaccination against tuberculosis by DNA injection. Nat Med 2: 888–892

Trinchieri G (1996) Interleukin-12 and its role in the generation of Th1 cells. Immunol Today 14: 335–337

Ward SG, Bacon K, Westwick J (1998) Chemokines and T lymphocytes: more than an attraction. Immunity 9: 1–11

Waisman A, Ruiz PJ, Hirschberg DL, Gelman A, Oksenberg JR, Brocke S, et al (1996) Suppressive vaccination with DNA encoding a variable region gene of the T-cell receptor prevents autoimmune encephalomyelitis and activates Th2 immunity. Nat Med 2: 899–905

Wildbaum G, Karin N (1999) Augmentation of natural immunity to a pro-inflammatory cytokine (TNF-alpha) by targeted DNA vaccine confers long-lasting resistance to experimental autoimmune encephalo-myelitis. Gene Ther 6: 1128–1138

Wildbaum G, Youssef S, Grabie N, Karin N (1998) Prevention of experimental autoimmune encephalomy-elitis by antibodies to interferon gamma inducing factor. J Immunol 161: 6368–6374

Wildbaum G, Westermann J, Maor G, Karin N (2000a) A targeted DNA vaccine encoding fas ligand defines its dual role in the regulation of experimental autoimmune encephalomyelitis. J Clin Invest 106: 671–679

Wildbaum G, Youssef S, Karin N (2000b) A targeted DNA vaccine augments the natural immune response to self TNF-alpha and suppresses ongoing adjuvant arthritis. J Immunol 165: 5860–5866

Yednock TA, Cannon C, Fritz LC, Sanchez MF, Steinman L, Karin N (1992) Prevention of experimental autoimmune encephalomyelitis by antibodies against alpha 4 beta 1 integrin. Nature 356: 63–66

Youssef S, Wildbaum G, Maor G, Lanir N, Gour-Lavie A, Grabie N, et al (1998) Long lasting protective immunity to experimental autoimmune encephalomyelitis following vaccination with naked DNA encoding C-C chemokines. J Immunol 161: 3870–3879

Youssef S, Wildbaum G, Karin N (1999) Prevention of experimental autoimmune encephalomyelitis by MIP-1alpha and MCP-1 naked DNA vaccines. J Autoimmun 13: 21–29

Youssef S, Maor G, Wildbaum G, Grabie N, Gour-Lavie A, Karin N (2000) C-C chemokine-encoding DNA vaccines enhance breakdown of tolerance to their gene products and treat ongoing adjuvant arthritis. J Clin Invest 106: 361–371

Immunosuppressive treatment of rheumatic diseases during pregnancy

Monika Østensen*

Department of Rheumatology and Clinical Immunology/Allergology,
University Hospital, Berne, Switzerland

Introduction

Rheumatic diseases have a predilection for the female sex and often become manifest during womens' childbearing years. The interaction of pregnancy and rheumatic diseases varies, some conditions benefit, others worsen in response to the immunological and hormonal alterations of pregnancy. Diseases which remain active during pregnancy may need drug treatment either for the benefit of the mother or in order to protect pregnancy and the fetus. Most often, immunosuppressive treatment is required in disorders associated with involvement of internal organs and autoimmune phenomena (Table 1).

This survey is based on a comprehensive search in the databases Embase, Medline, and Cochrane for the period 1960–2000 and presents data on the use of immunosuppressive and some cytostatic drugs during pregnancy. The interpretation of data is hampered by the scarcity of randomised, controlled trials in pregnant patients, the often small number of gestational drug exposures reported, and by the difficulty to ascribe observed negative events in the fetus or neonate to drugs, given the fact that the mother has an underlying disease. Furthermore, congenital malformations after drug exposure described in case reports have not always excluded other possible causes of anomalies like chromosomal aberrations.

Clearly, drug treatment in pregnancy has legal aspects and these are handled differently in different countries. Pharmaceutical companies who provide the drug information for the physician's desk reference take all precautions to avoid a law suit. Access to data of exposed human pregnancies is often difficult, since an uncomplicated pregnancy outcome most often is not reported, whereas a negative event is.

* Author's address: Department of Rheumatology and Clinical Immunology/Allergology, University Hospital, 3010 Bern, Switzerland.
E-mail: monika.oestensen@insel.ch

Table 1. Interaction between pregnancy and some common rheumatic diseases

Disease	Risk of major organ involvement during pregnancy	Indication for treatment during pregnancy	Immunosuppressives compatible with pregnancy[a]	Prevailing response of disease to pregnancy
Rheumatoid arthritis	rare	seldom	antimalarials, sulfasalazine, cyclosporine, azathioprine	improvement
Ankylosing spondylitis	no	often	sulfasalazine	active/aggravation
Juvenile chronic arthritis	no	seldom	antimalarials, sulfasalazine, cyclosporine, azathioprine	improvement
Systemic lupus erythematosus	renal, hematology, CNS	often	antimalarials, cyclosporine, azathioprine	aggravation
Connective-tissue diseases	renal, hematology, CNS	often	antimalarials, cyclosporine, azathioprine	active
Antiphospholipid syndrome	thromboembolic events	often	intravenous immunoglobulin	aggravation

[a] Monotherapy or combination therapy is often used together with prednisone

When choosing immunosuppression for a pregnant patient, considerations on the effect-to-risk ratio for mother and fetus are essential. The patient should be informed on what is documented and what is not known in regard to pregnancy. An approach which includes the patient as an active partner facilitates decision making.

Corticosteroids

Transplacental passage varies for the different corticosteroids according to their differing degree of inactivation by placenta hydroxylases. Inactivation is most effective for cortisol and prednisolone, but much less for dexamethasone and beta-methasone. Prednisolone or prednisone are therefore the most appropriate gluco-corticoids for the treatment of pregnant women, whereas dexamethasone and beta-methasone are reserved for fetal treatment, for example, to enhance fetal lung maturation prior to preterm delivery.

Maternal risks of prolonged and high doses (1–2 mg/kg/day) of corticosteroids are diabetes, elevated blood pressure, insomnia, depression, osteopenia, adrenal gland suppression, and susceptibility to infection. Premature rupture of membranes has been found increased in steroid-treated pregnancies (Petri 1998, Le Thi Huong et al. 2001).

Animal studies and early case reports of exposed human pregnancies reported cleft palate after first-trimester exposure to corticosteroids (Pinsky et al. 1965,

Fraser et al. 1995). Most studies including a limited number of patients and often without controls did not find evidence for an increased rate of congenital abnormalities in humans. In a survey of 457 exposed pregnancies in 1995, the incidence of cleft palate was found to be 2% versus 0.2% expected (Fraser et al. 1995). It was concluded that corticosteroids were not strong teratogens in humans. However, a recent metaanalysis of epidemiological studies found a significantly increased risk for oral clefts after first-trimester exposure to corticosteroids (Park-Wyllie et al. 2000).

Anecdotal reports on other adverse events of antenatal corticosteroid exposure are neonatal cataracts (Kraus 1975) and infection (Coté et al. 1974). Adrenal insufficiency with reduced cortisol levels in the neonate occurs infrequently, presumably in less than 4% of neonates (Kozlowska-Boszko et al. 1996). Maternal corticosteroid therapy does not induce general immunosuppression in the neonate.

The influence of corticosteroids on intrauterine growth has been controversial. The fact that an increased incidence of low-birth-weight babies was also found in corticosteroid-treated mothers without autoimmune or systemic disease suggests a drug effect (Scott 1977, Reinisch et al. 1978).

Comment. High doses like 1–2 mg/kg/day should be avoided in the first trimester. At a prednisone maintenance therapy at or below 15 mg/day only 5–10% of free prednisone will be present in maternal plasma. Calcium supplementation for prevention of osteopenia is advisable. Stress doses of corticosteroids must be given during delivery.

Immunosuppressive drugs

The immunosuppressive drugs antimalarials, sulphasalazine, azathioprine, and cyclosporine are used alone or in combination therapy with methotrexate and corticosteroids in the treatment of rheumatoid arthritis (RA), juvenile chronic arthritis (JCA), systemic lupus erythematosus (SLE), and other connective-tissue diseases. The use of combination therapies in pregnancy renders it difficult to ascribe adverse effects to a single drug unless a distinct fetal or neonatal syndrome is known to be induced by a particular drug. The risk for immunosuppression in the neonate exists, though the published literature shows this to be an infrequent event. Possible long-term effects of antenatal immunosuppression like induction of autoimmunity or malignancy and effects on reproductive function are largely unknown.

Antimalarial drugs

Daily doses of 250 mg of chloroquine or 200–400 mg of hydroxychloroquine are used to treat several rheumatic diseases like RA and SLE.

Chloroquine crosses the placenta and accumulates preferentially in melanin-containing structures in the fetal uveal tract and inner ear (Phillips-Howard et al. 1996). Abnormalities in the retina and the inner ear have been reported in two and three infants respectively exposed to higher than the recommended daily doses of chloroquine throughout pregnancy (Phillips-Howard et al. 1996, Hart et al. 1964).

In the rheumatic literature, for more than 100 pregnancies treated either with chloroquine (250 mg daily) or hydroxychloroquine (200–400 mg daily) during the first trimester no increase in congenital abnormalities was found (Buchanan et al. 1996, Levy et al. 1991, Parke 1988, Parke et al. 1996).

Comment. The long elimination half-life of antimalarials and their tendency to accumulate in melanin-containing tissues, including the retina, restricts their gestational use. Discontinuation of antimalarials in pregnant SLE patients may precipitate a flare with harmful consequences for mother and child. It seems therefore reasonable to continue antimalarials during pregnancy.

Sulphasalazine

Reports regarding the use of sulphasalazine during and after pregnancy originate exclusively from experience in patients with inflammatory-bowel disease.

More than 1300 pregnancies in patients with ulcerative colitis and nearly 800 in patients with Crohn's disease treated either with sulphasalazine alone or in combination with corticosteroids at some time during pregnancy have been reported (Mogadam et al. 1981, Willougby et al. 1980). No increase in birth defects, small for gestational-age babies, or an increase of pathological jaundice was detected.

Comment. Sulphasalazine is a dihydrofolate reductase inhibitor associated with a risk for congenital cardiovascular defects and oral clefts when given during the second and third month of gestation (Hernandez-Diaz et al. 2000). Folate supplementation given before and throughout pregnancy decreases this risk substantially. As neutropenia in a neonate occurred after high maternal doses, the daily dose should not exceed 2 g (Levi et al. 1988).

Azathioprine

Lacking the enzyme inosinate pyrophosphorylase, the fetal liver is unable to convert azathioprine to its active form. Therefore, the fetus should theoretically be protected from the effects of azathioprine and its active metabolite 6-mercaptopurine in early pregnancy (Alstead et al. 1990).

Accumulated data on pregnancies in renal allograft recipients or patients with SLE treated with corticosteroids and azathioprine found no predominant or frequent birth defect (Registration Committee 1980, Meehan et al. 1987, Ramsey-Goldman et al. 1993). In a European survey (Registration Committee 1980) on transplant recipients, birth anomalies were present in seven of 103 children. Mothers of abnormal babies had taken significantly higher doses of azathioprine (2.64 mg/kg versus 2.02 mg/kg) than those with healthy babies. Case reports have described congenital malformations and immunosuppression in several infants; however, a causal relationship to azathioprine has not been proven (Williamson et al. 1981). Fetal growth restriction has sometimes been related to the gestational use of azathioprine and corticosteroids (Scott 1977). The possible contribution of the underlying maternal disease is unclear.

Intrauterine exposure to azathioprine may occasionally cause slight suppression of the bone marrow as shown by decreased leucocyte counts and thrombocytopenia at birth (Davison et al. 1985). T cell development is enhanced in the newborn after antenatal azathioprine exposure, but at later ages no induction of autoimmunity or immundefiency is seen (Pilarski et al. 1994). Follow-up of children exposed antenatally showed normal development during infancy and into adolescence.

Comment. There is no indication for azathioprine in doses of 1.5–2 mg/kg/day to be a strong teratogen or to cause lasting immunosuppression in the neonate. Adjustment of the maternal leucocyte count during pregnancy by dose reduction avoids neonatal depression of hemopoiesis.

Cyclosporine

Cyclosporine is used primarily as an immunosuppressive drug to prevent rejection of organ transplantation. The efficacy of cyclosporine has been demonstrated in patients with RA and SLE whose conditions have not responded to conventional therapy.

More than 600 pregnancies exposed to cyclosporine for several weeks or throughout gestation have been reported (Cockburn et al. 1989, Armenti et al. 1994, Gaughan et al. 1996, Lamarque et al. 1997). The majority of the treated mothers were transplant recipients. Daily doses ranged from 1.4 to 14 mg/kg with a mean dose of 5 mg/kg. The observed rate of 3% of congenital malformations has not exceeded the rate reported in the general population, nor has any particular pattern of abnormalities emerged. Renal and liver functions were normal in 166 neonates exposed to cyclosporine in utero (Shaheen et al. 1993). Major problems of cyclosporine-treated pregnancies were prematurity (<37 weeks) in 40–46% and low birth weight (<2500 g) in 44–65% of cases. The contribution of the underlying maternal disorder is unclear.

Follow-up for 1 to 12 years of 175 children registered in the National Transplantation Pregnancy Register (U.S.A.) found normal development in 84% of offspring exposed to cyclosporine in utero (Stanley et al. 1999). The high incidence of prematurity was suspected to be involved in the mental developmental delay observed in 16% of the children. Since cyclosporine can induce autoimmunity in rodents after exposure in utero, several studies have addressed this issue in children of transplant recipients. Though T, B, and NK cell maturation and development can be impaired during the first year of life (Di Paolo 2000), a follow-up ranging from 0.5 to 9 years of age found normal immune function in 10 children exposed to cyclosporine throughout pregnancy (Pilarski et al. 1994).

Comment. There is no indication that cyclosporine is a human teratogen or that it causes autoimmunity in children exposed in utero.

Mycophenolate mofetil

Mycophenolate mofetil (Cellcept), an inhibitor of purine synthesis, has been successfully employed to prevent transplant rejection. As an immunosuppressive agent with a more pronounced effect on T and B cells, Cellcept has also been used for the treatment of immunological disorders like severe, refractory RA and lupus nephritis with some promising results.

In animal studies, treatment of pregnant rats and rabbits with 0.3 to 0.5 times the human doses have resulted in birth defects comprising the central nervous system and the cardiovascular and renal systems. Cellcept is not recommended to be used in women of fertile years without safe contraception. However, the concurrence of pregnancy during treatment with cellcept has occurred (Armenti et al. 1998). Published reports are not available, but data exist in the files of the company. By January 2001, 44 pregnancies under treatment with cellcept have been reported; however, the outcome is known only for 18 of these pregnancies. Thirteen deliveries resulted in healthy neonates. Abnormalities at birth were observed in five neonates, yet a causative role of cellcept could not be established.

Comment. Because of the very limited experience in human pregnancy, Cellcept is not recommended during pregnancy.

Cytotoxic drugs

Methotrexate

Low-dose weekly pulses of 5–20 mg of methotrexate (MTX) are widely used for inflammatory rheumatic diseases, either as monotherapy or in combination with other immunosuppressive drugs.

Transplacental passage of MTX has been demonstrated by detecting the drug and polyglutamates in cord blood and erythrocytes of one neonate (Schleunig et al. 1987).

MTX is a folic acid antagonist which impairs dihydrofolate reductase and interferes with the production of purines. Absolute or functional folic acid deficiency during early pregnancy will typically lead to neural tube defects in the offspring but can also induce other abnormalities. The congenital anomalies observed in animals and humans exposed to MTX in utero usually involved the central nervous system, cranial ossification, and the palate. Three infants exposed to MTX during the first trimester had multiple cranial anomalies. In seven cases, MTX had been given during late pregnancy; six normal children were born and one child had pancytopenia (Doll et al. 1989).

Reviewing the rheumatology literature of first-trimester exposure to once weekly doses of 20 mg of MTX or less, disclosed 20 pregnancies (Østensen et al. 2000). In the pregnancies not terminated electively, four (22%) ended in miscarriage, and of the 12 which proceeded to delivery, one child (8%) was born with the "aminopterin syndrome". Birth weights of the full-term infants were within normal range. A follow-up ranging from 0.1 to 16.7 years of seven of the children revealed no developmental or other serious health problems.

Comment. MTX is contraindicated during pregnancy and should be prescribed to fertile women only under the cover of safe contraception. Due to the possibility that active metabolites remain in cells or tissues for about two months after cessation of therapy, conception should be postponed until three months after withdrawal of the drug. Folate supplementation should be continued antenatally and throughout pregnancy.

Cyclophosphamide

Severe forms of systemic rheumatic diseases like SLE, JCA, and RA are sometimes treated with cyclophosphamide either orally or, as in lupus nephritis, as intravenous pulse therapy.

Cyclophosphamide is an alkylating agent which is teratogenic in all animal species studied (Mirkes 1985). The effect on human pregnancy seems to be unpredictable as both normal children and children with congenital anomalies have been reported. The picture is complicated by concurrent treatment with other cytotoxic agents or radiation therapy in pregnant patients with malignancies. Birth defects have been reported in human fetuses after first-trimester exposure to cyclophosphamide with facial, skin, musculoskeletal, and visceral organ anomalies, growth retardation, and developmental delay during childhood (Briggs et al. 1998). Intravenous cyclophosphamide therapy given during the first trimester in seven pregnancies of six women with lupus nephritis resulted in 2 miscarriages, 1 elective termination of pregnancy, 2 children with multiple anomalies, 1 child with short arms and legs, and 1 healthy child.

Comment. Cyclophosphamide is a human teratogen. Safe contraception is necessary when fertile women are treated with the drug. Attempts of conception should be delayed until three months after cessation of therapy.

New immunosuppressive drugs

In the years 1999 and 2000 leflunomide and the tumor necrosis factor alpha (TNF-α) antagonists infliximab and etanercept were registered for the treatment of RA and the TNF-α antagonists also for Crohn's disease.

Leflunomide

Studies in pregnant rats and rabbits with doses equivalent to human doses have found teratogenicity and fetotoxicity of leflunomide. Both skeletal and central nervous system malformations have been observed. In addition, increased embryolethality and reduced fetal weight were noted.

One abstract has reported the occurrence of pregnancy during treatment with leflunomide. Of the 25 pregnancies exposed, 22 were interrupted, three pregnancies went to delivery, but details of neonatal health are not known (Brent 1998).

Comment. Leflunomide is contraindicated during pregnancy and women of childbearing potential should be started on the drug only under safe contraception. Due to its long half-life and protracted elimination from plasma, leflunomide must be withdrawn before a planned pregnancy and conception first attempted after successful elimination of the drug by cholestyramine or active charcoal (Brent 2001).

TNF-α antagonists

Pharmacological TNF-α inhibition can be achieved by monoclonal antibodies (infliximab) or by soluble TNF-α receptors (TNF-R) (etanercept). Thus far, there are few reports on completed human pregnancies exposed to TNF-α inhibitors.

Soluble TNF-R cross the placenta and gain access to the fetal circulation in mice but do not interrupt pregnancy or impair fetal development (Goroir et al. 1992). Pregnancy studies in rats and rabbits with 60–100 times the human dose of etanercept did not find teratogenicity or fetotoxicity of the drug. Pregnancy proceeds normally in TNF-α knockout mice.

No embryo- or fetotoxicity was noted in mice treated with an antibody analogue to the human monoclonal antibody. In an abstract, exposure to infliximab has been reported for 42 pregnancies (Katz et al. 2001). No increase in negative pregnancy outcome or congenital abnormalities has been reported for the 35 pregnancies followed to term.

Comment. Due to a lack of sufficient human data, the use of etanercept or infliximab during pregnancy is not recommended.

Intravenous immunoglobulin

Intravenous immunoglobulin is applied in serious autoimmune conditions when other treatment has failed. Experience in pregnant patients stems from treatment of severe idiopathic thrombopenic purpura, recurrent abortion, antiphospholipid syndrome and adult Still's disease. In rheumatology, the antiphospholipid syndrome has been the main indication for treatment of pregnant patients with the aim to prevent miscarriage. Whereas case reports and uncontrolled studies reported favorable effects on pregnancy outcome in the antiphospholipid syndrome (Harris et al. 1998), the only controlled study of 16 pregnant patients showed no effect of intravenous immunoglobulin (Branch et al. 2000). Maternal and fetal tolerance to intravenous immunoglobulin has been good.

Conclusion

Immunosuppressive treatment during pregnancy should control maternal disease activity and ensure a successful pregnancy outcome. Corticosteroids are often efficient in controlling disease flares. However, due to an increased risk of oral clefts, high doses should be avoided in the first trimester. In case of active SLE or RA, treatment with antimalarials or sulphasalazine may continue during pregnancy. Insufficient data exist for treatment of pregnant patients with new immunosuppressives like mycophenolate mofetil and the TNF-inhibitors. The severity of the disease under treatment decides whether continuation of one of these drugs is justified. Prophylactic withdrawal of drugs before pregnancy is mandatory for leflunomide and the cytotoxic agents methotrexate and cyclophosphamide. Folate supplementation before and during pregnancy is important when folic acid antagonists like sulphasalazine and methotrexate have been prescribed. Prepregnancy counselling and careful monitoring during pregnancy help to tailor necessary drug treatment for the benefit of mother and child.

References

Alstead EM, Ritchie JK, Lennard-Jones JE, Farthing MJG, Clark ML (1990) Safety of azathioprine in pregnancy in inflammatory bowel disease. Gastroenterology 99: 443–446

Armenti VT, Ahlswede KM, Ahlswede BA, Jarrell BE, Moritz MJ, Burke JF (1994) National transplantation pregnancy registry: outcomes of 154 pregnancies in cyclosporine-treated female kidney transplant recipients. Transplantation 57: 502–506

Armenti VT, Moritz MJ, Davison JM (1998) Drug safety issues in pregnancy following transplantation and immunosuppression. Drug Saf 19: 219–232

Branch DW, Peaceman AM, Druzin M et al. (2000) A multicenter, placebo-controlled pilot study of intravenous immune globuline treatment of antiphospholipid syndrome during pregnancy. Am J Obstet Gynecol 182: 122–127

Briggs GG, Freeman RK, Yaffe SJ (1998) Drugs in pregnancy and lactation, 5th edn. Williams & Wilkins, Baltimore, pp 272c–279c

Brent RL (1998) Leflunomide as an example of a modern approach to product labelling for reproductive effects: a category X drug based on pharmacokinetic data. Teratology 58: 445

Brent RL (2001) Teratogen update: reproductive risks of leflunomide (Arava), a pyrimidine synthesis inhibitor: counseling women taking leflunomide before or during pregnancy and men taking leflunomide who are contemplating fathering a child. Teratology 63: 106–112

Buchanan NMM, Toubi E, Khamashta KE, Lima F, Kerslake S, Hughes GRV (1996) Hydoxychloroquine and lupus pregnancy: review of a series of 36 cases. Ann Rheum Dis 55: 486–488

Cockburn I, Krupp P, Monka C (1989) Present experience of Sandimmun in pregnancy. Transplant Proc 21: 3730–3732

Coté CJ, Meuwissen HG, Pickering RJ (1974) Effects on the neonate of prednisone and azathioprine administered to the mother during pregnancy. J Pediatr 85: 324–328

Davison JM, Dellagrammatikos H, Parkin JM (1985) Maternal azathioprine therapy and depressed haemopoiesis in the babies of renal allograft patients. Br J Obst Gynecol 92: 233–239

Di Paolo S, Schena A, Morrone LF, Manfredi G, Stallone G, Derosa C, Procino A, Schena FP (2000). Immunologic evaluation during the first year of life of infants born to cyclosporine-treated female kidney transplant recipients. Transplantation 69: 2049–2054

Doll CD, Ringenberg QS, Yarbro JW (1989) Antineoplastic agents and pregnancy. Semin Oncol 16: 337–346

Fraser FC, Sajoo A (1985) Teratogenic potential of corticosteroids in humans. Teratology 51: 45–46

Gaughan WJ, Moritz MJ, Radomski JS, Burke JF Jr, Armenti VT (1996) National Transplantation Pregnancy Registry: report on outcomes in cyclosporine-treated female kidney transplant recipients with an interval from transplant to pregnancy of greater than five years. Am J Kidney Dis 28: 266–269

Goroir BP, Peppel K, Silva M, Beutler B (1992) The biosynthesis of tumor necrosis factor during pregnancy: studies with a CAT reporter transgene and TNF inhibitors. Eur Cytokine Network 3: 533–537

Harris EN, Pierangeli SS (1998) Utilization of intravenous immunoglobulin therapy to treat recurrent pregnancy loss in the antiphospholipid syndrome: a review. Scand J Rheumatol (Suppl) 107: 97–102

Hart CN, Naunton RF (1964) The ototoxicity of chloroquine phosphate. Arch Otolaryngol Head Neck Surg 80: 407–412

Hernandez-Diaz S, Werler MM, Walker AM, Mitchell AA (2000) Folic acid antagonists during pregnancy and the risk of birth defects. N Eng J Med 343: 1608–1614

Katz JA, Lichtenstein GR, Keenan GF, Healy DE, Jacobs SJ (2001) Outcome of pregnancy in women receiving remicade (Infliximab) for the treatment of Crohn's disease or rheumatoid arthritis. American Gastroenterological Association, Digestive Disease Week, Atlanta, April 2001, Abstract 366

Kozlowska-Boszko B, Soluch L, Rybus J, Lao M, Durlik M, Gaciong Z (1996) Does chronic glucosteroid therapy in pregnant renal allograft recipients affect cortisol levels in neonates? Transplant Proc 28: 3490–3491

Kraus AM (1975) Congenital cataract and maternal steroid injection. J Pediatr Ophthalmol Strabismus 12: 107–108

Lamarque V, Leleu MF, Monka C, Krupp P (1997) Analysis of 629 pregnancy outcomes in transplant recipients treated with Sandimmun. Transplant Proc 29: 2480

Le Thi Huong D, Wechsler B, Bletry O, Vauthier-Brouzes D, Lefebvre G, Piette JC (2001) A study of 75 pregnancies in patients with antiphospholipid syndrome. J Rheumatol 28: 2025–2030

Levi S, Liberman M, Levi AJ, Bjarnason I (1988) Reversible congenital neutropenia associated with maternal sulphasalazine therapy (letter). Eur J Pediatr 148: 174–175

Levy M, Buskila D, Gladman DD, Urowitz MB, Koren G (1991) Pregnancy outcome following first trimester exposure to chloroquine. Am J Perinatol 8: 174–178

Meehan RT, Dorsey JK (1987) Pregnancy among patients with systemic lupus erythematosus receiving immunosuppressive therapy. J Rheumatol 14: 252–258

Mirkes PE (1985) Cyclophosphamide teratogenesis: a review. Teratog Carcinog Mutagen 5: 75–88

Mogadam M, Dobbins WO, Korelitz BI, Ahmed SW (1981) Pregnancy in inflammatory bowel disease: effect of sulphasalazine and corticosteroids on fetal outcome. Gastroenterology 80: 72–76

Østensen M, Hartmann H, Salvesen K (2000) Low dose weekly methotrexate in early pregnancy: a case series and review of the literature. J Rheumatol 27: 1872–1875

Parke AL (1988) Antimalarial drugs, systemic lupus erythematosus and pregnancy. J Rheumatol 15: 607–610

Parke AL, West B (1996) Hydoxychloroquine in pregnant patients with systemic lupus erythematosus. J Rheumatol 23: 1715–1718

Park-Wyllie L, Mazzotta P, Pastuszak A, Moretti ME, Beique L, Hunnisett L, Friesen MH, Jacobson S, Kasapinovic S, Chang D, Diav-Citrin O, Chitayat D, Nulman I, Einarson TR, Koren G (2000) Birth defects after maternal exposure to corticosteroids: prospective cohort study and meta-analysis of epidemiological studies. Teratology 62: 385–392

Petri M (1998) Pregnancy and SLE. Baillieres Clin Rheumatol 12: 449–476

Phillips-Howard PA, Wood D (1996) The safety of antimalarial drugs in pregnancy. Drug Saf 14: 131–145

Pilarski LM, Yacyshyn BR, Lazarovits AI (1994) Analysis of peripheral blood lymphocyte populations and immune function from children exposed to cyclosporine or to azathioprine in utero. Transplantation 57: 133–144

Pinsky L, DiGeorge AM (1965) Cleft palate in the mouse: a teratogenic index of glucocorticoid potency. Science 147: 402–403

Ramsey-Goldman R, Mientus JM, Kutzer JE, Mulvihill JJ, Medsger TA (1993) Pregnancy outcome in women with systemic lupus erythematosus treated with immunosuppressive drugs. J Rheumatol 20: 1152–1157

Registration Committee of the European Dialysis and Transplant Association (1980) Successful pregnancies in women treated by dialysis and kidney transplantation. Br J Obstet Gynaecol 87: 839–845

Reinisch JM, Simon NG (1978) Prenatal exposure to prednisone in humans and animals retards intrauterine growth. Science 202: 436–438

Schleuning M, Clemm C (1987) Chromosomal aberrations in a newborn whose mother received cytotoxic treatment during pregnancy. N Engl J Med 317: 1666–1667

Scott JR (1977) Fetal growth retardation associated with maternal administration of immunosuppressives. Am J Obstet Gynecol 128: 668–676

Shaheen FAM, Al-Sulaiman MH, Al-Khader AA (1993) Long-term nephrotoxicity after exposure to cyclosporine in utero. Transplantation 56: 224–225

Stanley CW, Gottlieb R, Zager R, Eisenberg J, Richmond R, Moritz MJ, Armenti VT (1999) Developmental well-being in offspring of women receiving post-renal transplant. Transplant Proc 31: 241–242

Williamson RA, Karp LE (1981) Azathioprine teratogenicity: review of the literature and case report. Obstet Gynecol 58: 247–250

Willoughby CP, Truelove SC (1980) Ulcerative colitis and pregnancy. Gut 21: 469–474

Persistence of maternal and fetal cells in autoimmune diseases

Anne M. Stevens[1,2,*], **J. Lee Nelson**[1,3], and **Nathalie Lambert**[1]

[1]Program in Human Immunogenetics, Fred Hutchinson Cancer Research Center, [2]Division of Rheumatology, Immunology, and Infectious Diseases, Department of Pediatrics, University of Washington, Children's Hospital and Regional Medical Center, and [3]Division of Rheumatology, Department of Medicine, University of Washington, Seattle, Washington, U.S.A.

Introduction

It has long been known that maternal proteins are transported to the fetus during pregnancy. Maternal antibodies provide immunity for the newborn infant during the first six months of life. Only recently with the advent of ultrasensitive DNA detection techniques has it been established that there is bidirectional traffic of not only antibodies but also cells. The term "chimerism" is used when one individual harbors cells from another individual; "microchimerism" refers to low levels of chimerism. When cells traffic between fetus and mother during pregnancy and persist, maternal and fetal microchimerism results. Chronic graft-versus-host disease (GVHD) is a condition of chimerism that shares clinical characteristics with some autoimmune diseases. Human leukocyte antigen (HLA) class II genes are known to be important both in autoimmune disease and in GVHD. When considered together, these observations led to the hypothesis that microchimerism and HLA genes of host and nonhost cells are involved in autoimmune disease. Sources of nonhost cells include cells transferred during pregnancy (maternal and fetal), a twin or unrecognized lost twin, or a blood transfusion. By this hypothesis, women who have been pregnant have an increased risk of autoimmune disease because they have two sources of microchimerism: maternal and fetal. Studies of systemic sclerosis, primary biliary cirrhosis, Sjögren's syndrome, pruritic eruption of pregnancy, myositis, neonatal lupus, and thyroid disease have both lent support and raised doubts about the role of microchimerism in autoimmune disease.

* Authors' address: Immunogenetics D2-100, Fred Hutchinson Cancer Research Center, 1100 Fairview Avenue North, Seattle, WA 98109-1024, U.S.A.

Microchimerism from pregnancy and from other sources

Fetal cells pass into the maternal circulation during normal human pregnancy. Evidence for fetal cells in the mother's circulation has been described as early as 4 to 5 weeks of gestation (Thomas et al. 1994). Bianchi et al. (1996) described persistent fetal microchimerism in the peripheral circulation of healthy women many years after pregnancy completion. Women were studied who had given birth to sons. Peripheral blood was tested for male DNA after sorting for cells expressing CD34 and CD38, markers for progenitor cells. 6 of the 8 women tested had male DNA in the progenitor cell population and 1 of 5 women tested had male DNA within her T lymphocyte population. Thus, persistent fetal microchimerism commonly occurs after normal pregnancy.

Cell traffic during pregnancy is now known to be bidirectional, with maternal cells also passing into the fetal circulation. A number of early reports described persistent maternal microchimerism in immunodeficient infants, where the allogeneic maternal cells can cause GVHD (Pollack et al. 1982). By fluorescence in situ hybridization (FISH) with probes to the X and Y chromosomes, maternal cells were found in 14% of cord blood samples from male infants (Hall et al. 1995). Maternal cells were found in both the $CD8^+$ and $CD34^+$ subsets. In reports using more sensitive PCR-based assays, maternal DNA was found in 24–100% of cord blood samples (Petit et al. 1995; Lo et al. 1996, 2000). Maternal DNA has also been reported in the fetal circulation as early as 13 weeks in blood samples taken prior to elective terminations (Lo et al. 2000). Lo et al. (2000) developed quantitative techniques to study bidirectional traffic and found mother-to-fetus transfer was common, though it was less frequent than from fetus to mother and at lower quantities. Maternal cells have been estimated at a rate of 0.02–5% in cord blood (Hall et al. 1995, Petit et al. 1997, Lo et al. 2000). Three studies have found that maternal microchimerism can persist throughout childhood and into adult life in immunocompetent progeny (Maloney et al. 1999, Artlett et al. 2000a, Reed et al. 2000).

Other sources of microchimerism include cells from a twin (De Moor et al. 1988, Victor et al. 2000) or from a blood transfusion (Lee et al. 1999). Fetal microchimerism is assumed to occur after pregnancies that end in miscarriage or induced abortion, because fetal cells have been found early in normal pregnancies. A large amount of fetal DNA has been described in the circulation of women following elective termination (Bianchi et al. 2001).

Chimerism in transplantation

After hematopoietic stem cell transplantation a patient becomes chimeric. Chronic GVHD can occur as a complication of stem cell transplantation. Chronic GVHD has clinical similarities with systemic sclerosis (SSc), primary biliary cirrhosis (PBC), Sjögren's syndrome, and sometimes has features of systemic lupus and myositis (Table 1). The majority of patients with chronic GVHD have antinuclear antibodies (Rouquette-Gally et al. 1987). There are, however, clear differences. The pulmonary disease of GVHD is usually obstructive, whereas in SSc it is restrictive. Renal

Table 1. Comparison of the clinical aspects of chronic GVHD with autoimmune diseases

Clinical aspect	Occurrence in:	
	autoimmune disease	GVHD
Scleroderma	very common	very common
Myositis	common	rare, but reported
Sicca syndrome	common	common
Hepatic	common	common
Gastrointestinal	common	common
Pulmonary	restrictive	obstructive
Renal	common	not increased
Raynaud's	very common	not increased
SSc antibodies	common	reported
Antinuclear antibodies	common	common

disease is seen in SSc but is rarely part of GVHD. Finally, in GVHD the foreign cells make up the majority of the hematopoietic population, whereas in SSc foreign fetal or maternal cells are in the minority.

Fetal microchimerism in human disease

Fetal microchimerism has been found in autoimmune conditions resembling GVHD, with multiple organs as targets (Fig. 1): SSc, PBC of the liver, pruritic eruption of pregnancy, sicca syndrome (Sjögren's disease), and thyroiditis.

The first description of microchimerism in an autoimmune disease was a quantitative study of fetal microchimerism in women with SSc compared to healthy controls (Nelson et al. 1998). The study was prospective and blinded. Women with SSc were studied who had given birth to at least one son prior to disease onset. Controls were healthy women with at least one son. Women with sons were studied for the technical reason that it enabled the use of a single assay that detected male DNA in a female host. By assaying 10 or more aliquots of DNA isolated from whole blood from each subject, the number of male DNA cell equivalents in $16\,cm^3$ of blood was estimated. The results indicated a range of male DNA cell equivalents among healthy controls of 0 to 2 per $16\,cm^3$, with a mean of 0.38. In contrast, the range was 0 to 61 with a mean of 11.1 in women with SSc ($P = 0.0007$). Some SSc patients had levels of male DNA that were higher than that found in women who are currently pregnant with a male fetus, although these patients had given birth to their sons decades previously. Other investigators used a nested PCR assay to study DNA extracted from skin biopsies and peripheral blood (Artlett et al. 1998). Male DNA was found in 32 of 69 peripheral blood mononuclear cell (PBMC) samples and 11 of 19 skin biopsy samples from women with SSc. Male cells were seen in some skin biopsy samples by FISH. A weakness of this study was that pregnancy histories were incomplete (known for only 2 of 94 subjects studied for peripheral microchimerism), preventing a direct comparison of controls

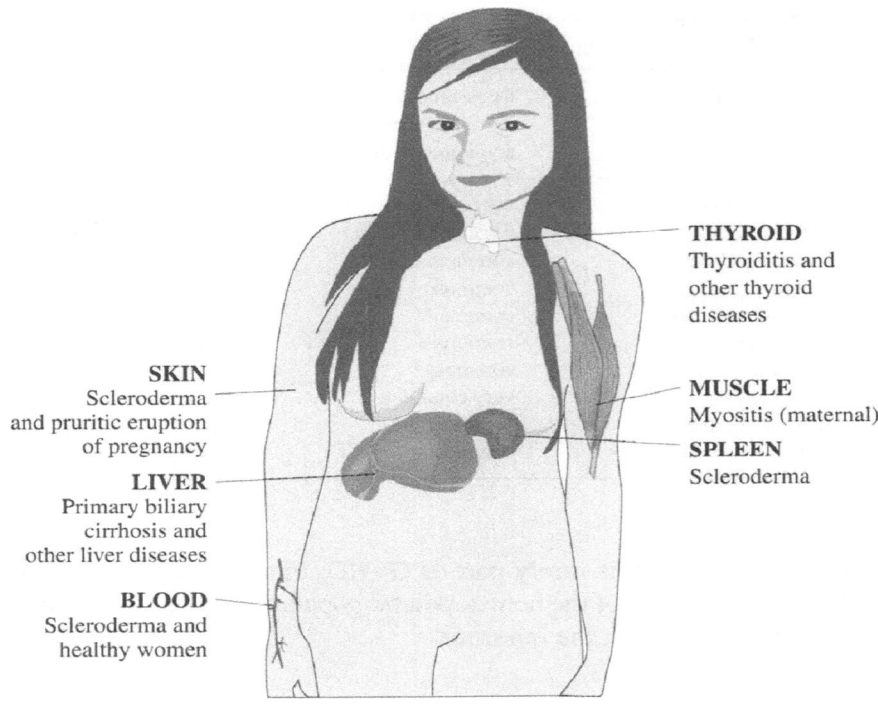

Fig. 1. Fetal and maternal microchimerism has been found in multiple target organs

to patients. Women without sons would have been counted as negative for fetal cells when they were actually uninformative cases. Moreover, microchimerism in T lymphocytes was reported in women with SSc, but no controls were assayed for comparison. Subsequent studies confirmed the earlier report by Bianchi that persistent fetal microchimerism is common among T lymphocytes (and also among B cells, NK cells, and monocytes) in both women with SSc and healthy women (Evans et al. 1999). Other studies have examined persistent fetal microchimerism in women with SSc with variable results (Murata et al. 1999, Artlett et al. 2000b, Ichikawa et al. 2001).

Fetal microchimerism has been investigated in a number of studies of patients with PBC. The first report of PBC patients described male fetal DNA detected in liver biopsies of women with PBC and in control patients with other, non-autoimmune liver conditions (Tanaka et al. 2000). Male DNA was found with approximately the same frequency in the two groups. Quantitative levels of male DNA were somewhat greater in PBC patients compared to disease controls, but the difference was not significant. Other reports also described fetal DNA detected in DNA extracted from liver biopsies and peripheral blood cells, with no significant difference in PBC patients compared to controls (Corpechot et al. 2000, Invernizzi et al. 2000). In a larger study, a different group (Fanning et al. 2000) found male cells by in situ hybridization in the livers of 42% of 19 PBC patients compared to none of the 20 control livers. In this study and a previous, smaller study (Rubbia-

Brandt et al. 1999), no male cells were found in the inflammatory infiltrates surrounding the damaged bile ducts.

Other studies have examined patients with Sjögren's syndrome. Two studies used nested PCR amplification to test for male DNA in total PBMC and in PBMC enriched for CD34 (stem cells) and found no significant difference between patients and healthy controls (Miyashita et al. 2000, Toda et al. 2001). In a carefully conducted study of skin biopsies from women with pruritic eruption of pregnancy that included microdissection of epidermal and dermal layers followed by testing for male DNA, women with the disease carried male DNA (Aractingi et al. 1998). Control biopsies from women pregnant with male fetuses who had other types of rashes or no rashes (caesarean section scars) and from women pregnant with female fetuses had no detectable male DNA.

Fetal microchimerism is of interest in autoimmune thyroiditis because of its increased incidence in the postpartum period. In one study (Klintschar et al. 2001), DNA was extracted from female thyroid specimens of women with and without sons and PCR amplification conducted for male DNA. Positive results were found in women who had sons, and an increased frequency of microchimerism was found in DNA extracted from thyroids affected by Hashimoto's disease compared to nodular goiter. In another study (Srivatsa et al. 2001), female thyroid specimens were studied by FISH with probes to the X and Y chromosomes to identify male cells. Male cells were detected significantly more often in disease-affected than disease-free thyroid specimens from autopsy samples. Male cells, however, were not limited to patients with thyroiditis, sometimes being found in patients with adenoma, multinodular goiter, and thyroid carcinoma. These two studies suggest fetal microchimerism may affect thyroid health of the mother but at the same time clearly raise questions regarding the role of microchimerism in autoimmune disease, given the detection of microchimerism in other thyroid conditions.

Fetal-maternal HLA relationships in human disease

Microchimerism may contribute to disease pathogenesis within the context of specific factors, i.e., exogenous triggers and particular human leukocyte antigen (HLA) genes. HLA genes could potentially be involved in at least three ways: the specific HLA allele of host cells, the specific HLA allele of the nonhost cells, and/or the HLA relationship of the two cell populations, all of which could contribute to disease risk. HLA molecules play a central role in an individual's ability to distinguish "self" from "foreign" and/or "danger". HLA molecules are of importance to stem cell transplantation success and HLA class II molecules, especially DR and DQ, are known to be associated with autoimmune diseases (Morrow et al. 1999). Thus, insights from transplantation chimerism contributed to the hypothesis that microchimerism and HLA relationships of host and nonhost cells are involved in spontaneously occurring autoimmune diseases (Nelson 1996). Initial studies of microchimerism and HLA relationships of host and nonhost cells examined SSc. Particular HLA-DRB1 alleles are associated with increased risk of SSc (Morrow et al. 1999). The specific HLA allele of the child could also be a contributory factor; as another study found, the strongest risk factor for a woman to have persistent fetal microchimerism among T lymphocytes was the particular HLA allele of the child. Specifically, DQA1*0501 has been associated with SSc (Arnett et al. 1996, Lambert et al. 2000a) and with fetal microchimerism (Lambert et al. 2000b, Reed et al. 2000).

The hypothesis regarding microchimerism and risk of autoimmune disease includes the postulate that the HLA relationships of host and nonhost cells are important in determining pathogenic potential of long-term persistent microchimerism (Nelson 1996). Widely HLA-disparate cells presumably could easily be identified as different from "self". HLA similarity could be detrimental because nonhost cells that are very similar but not entirely identical to the host could be tolerated by the host but later become activated and recognize the host as foreign. The initial study of fetal microchimerism examined risk of disease for the mother, so that HLA compatibility was examined from the mother's perspective. Two types of HLA relationships result in compatibility from the mother's perspective: (1) the child is HLA identical to the mother and (2) the child is HLA homozygous. In the first case, HLA compatibility is bidirectional. In the second case, compatibility is unidirectional. Whereas the mother would not recognize the child's cells as foreign, from the child's perspective the mother's HLA would appear foreign.

Maternal-fetal HLA compatibility was examined in women with SSc. HLA alleles were determined for 21 SSc patients and 32 control healthy women and all of their children (Nelson et al. 1998). The population studied for HLA alleles only partially overlapped with that studied for microchimerism. This was because at the time the only assay available to quantitatively assess microchimerism was one that identified male DNA, which therefore could only be used for women who had sons. On the other hand, the HLA studies required that all children participate, because the hypothesis tested was that any birth that is HLA compatible increases SSc risk. Therefore noninclusion of a child would be a methodological error with potential misclassification of a patient or control. Prior birth of a child who was compatible for HLA-DRB1 was associated with an almost ninefold increased risk of subsequent SSc in the mother, with risk increasing to 19 times if the child was HLA compatible due to homozygosity. Additional risk associated with homozygosity is of interest in light of the observation that recipients of blood transfusions from family members who are HLA compatible due to homozygosity are at increased risk of fatal GVHD (McMilin and Johnson 1993). HLA compatibility was also increased for DQA1 and DQB1 among SSc patients compared to controls, but the association was weaker than for DRB1. No association was observed for HLA-A, -B, or -C. The number of families studied for both microchimerism and HLA alleles was not sufficient to determine whether HLA-DRB1 compatibility correlated with quantitatively greater levels of fetal microchimerism.

Maternal microchimerism in human disease

Fetal cells may be a factor in the development of autoimmune disease in parous women, contributing to the gender preference of these diseases. However, men, children, and women who have never been pregnant also develop autoimmune disease. In these patients, maternal cells may be involved. It has long been known that maternal cells can engraft into immunodeficient infants and can potentially cause a GVHD-like disease (Pollack et al. 1982). Microchimerism has been postulated to play a role in SLE by Mullinax et al. (1993), who proposed chimerism as the explanation for the development of SLE in a patient who received in utero exchange transfusions. Another reason to consider maternal microchimerism in some cases of SLE is because a recognized experimental model of SLE is created by the introduction of parental cells into progeny (Gleichmann et al. 1982, Portanova et al. 1988). In this major histocompatibility complex antigen-dependent model, antinuclear antibodies are produced in large quantities and fatal immune complex glomerulonephritis develops, similar to spontaneously occurring SLE. Moreover, chronic GVHD after human stem cell transplantation can have features of SLE, including autoantibodies, neutropenia, and thrombocytopenia.

Persistent maternal microchimerism was recently described in the peripheral blood of a limited number of SSc patients and also in some healthy normals (Maloney et al. 1999). Addressing the HLA compatibility issue, a study purported to describe HLA compatibility of either the mother or the child as a risk factor for SSc (Artlett et al. 1997). Unfortunately, it is not possible to draw conclusions from this study because of several methodological problems. These include the use of patients with another HLA-associated disease as controls, inclusion of women for whom only some children were studied, and not considering the different HLA class II loci as nonindependent variables, although there is strong linkage disequilibrium of the DRB1, DQA1, and DQB1 genes. In a study that determined HLA alleles of men with SSc and their mothers, HLA compatibility of the mother did not differ from control men and mothers (Lambert et al. 2000a).

Juvenile idiopathic myositis is another autoimmune disease in which maternal cells may be involved. A mouse model of parental splenocyte transfusion results in myositis along with the SLE syndrome (Gelpi et al. 1994). Maternal microchimerism was recently investigated in children with juvenile dermatomyositis. One of the studies was particularly strong in design in that unaffected siblings were used as controls (Reed et al. 2000). 13 of 15 juvenile dermatomyositis patients had maternal microchimerism in peripheral blood samples, compared to 5 of 35 unaffected siblings (P < 0.0001). Maternal cells were detected in muscle tissue of 12 of 15 patients compared to 2 of 10 controls (P = 0.005). In a concurrent report (Artlett et al. 2000), ten male patients with probable or definite juvenile idiopathic inflammatory myopathy and ten controls with noninflammatory muscle diseases were studied for maternal microchimerism. Similarly, maternal microchimerism was significantly higher in patients compared to controls both in peripheral blood and in muscle biopsies. Maternal cells have also been found in the tissues of neonatal lupus patients who have died of congenital heart block (Stevens et al. 2001a).

Maternal microchimerism is found frequently in the absence of autoimmune disease in children and adults, suggesting that maternal cells alone do not cause disease. Maternal cells have been detected in the thymus of immunocompetent children (Stevens et al. 2001b). Likewise, in utero stem cell transplantation leads to permanent chimerism but not autoimmune disease (Victor 1998). Long-term effects of maternal microchimerism would not necessarily be expected to be the same as those of fetal microchimerism because long-lasting tolerance might be anticipated for maternal cells that passed into the fetus early in development, when the fetal immune system is just developing self-recognition. Issues such as timing during gestation, quantity and type of maternal cell exposure, and HLA genes could influence whether or not maternal cells that persist in the neonate and adult have pathogenic potential.

Whether or not microchimerism plays a role in disease pathogenesis remains to be determined. Studies thus far have demonstrated increased prevalence and increased levels of fetal microchimerism in autoimmune conditions, which could be interpreted to mean that fetal cells are actively triggering disease. Alternatively, fetal cells could be a secondary phenomenon, proliferating and increasing in numbers along with the host immune system in inflammatory conditions. The association of DRB1 compatibility of a previously born child with increased risk of SSc in the mother, however, argues against this interpretation. The most persuasive argument for a role in disease pathogenesis has been put forward by elegant studies in an experimental model described by Christner et al. (2000). In a series of experiments the investigators created a model of SSc by injecting a known SSc-associated agent, vinyl chloride, into mice that had been pregnant multiple times. Following administration of vinyl chloride, increased levels of fetal microchimerism were found accompanied by pathologic changes in skin and internal organs in mice that had been crossbred. Virgin mice had no detectable microchimerism and no pathology after vinyl chloride injections. Investigators also reported markedly enlarged spleens in the mice, an observation of further interest in light of a subsequent study of human autopsy specimens that the highest concentration of fetal cells in women with SSc is in the spleen (Johnson et al. 2001).

Concluding remarks

Allogeneic maternal and fetal cells can persist indefinitely in the blood and tissues of their new host. Microchimerism may be involved in the development of autoimmune disease. Fetal and maternal cells have been found in some studies to be increased in autoimmune patients compared to healthy controls, particularly when careful quantitative techniques have been used (Tables 2 and 3). In the child, the presence of maternal cells during early development could influence the selection of T lymphocytes recognizing self versus nonself, altering the T cell receptor repertoire. This could potentially lead to altered susceptibility to specific infections or to reactivity to self-antigens in the context of self or maternal HLA molecules.

Microchimerism is also found frequently in healthy controls. Thus, the phenomenon of microchimerism may have beneficial as well as detrimental effects on the mother and the child. One potential beneficial effect is the pregnancy-induced remission of rheumatoid arthritis. Arthritis amelioration during pregnancy was previously found to occur significantly more often in the context of fetal-maternal HLA disparity (Nelson et al. 1993). The protective effect of pregnancy on breast cancer risk (Lambe et al. 1994) also raises the interesting question of whether microchimerism could play a beneficial role in prevention of malignancy. Finally, the presence of fetal cells in the woman's circulation may

Table 2. Fetal cells in human diseases

Disease	Detection technique	Sample	Increase in cell number	Reference(s)
PBC	nested PCR	tissue	no	Tanaka et al. 2000
	PCR	tissue	no	Corpechot et al. 2000
	PCR	tissue	no	Invernizzi et al. 2000
	FISH	tissue	yes	Fanning et al. 2000
	FISH	tissue	no	Rubbia-Brandt et al. 1999
Thyroiditis	PCR	tissue	yes	Klintschar et al. 2001
	FISH	tissue	yes	Srivatsa et al. 2001
Systemic sclerosis	direct PCR	blood	yes	Nelson et al. 1998
	nested PCR, FISH	blood, tissues	yes	Artlett et al. 1998, 2000
	FISH	tissues	yes	Johnson et al. 2001
	PCR	blood	yes	Evans et al. 1999
		blood	no	Ichikawa et al. 2001
Sjögren's syndrome	nested PCR	blood, CD34$^+$	no	Toda et al. 2001
	nested PCR	PBMC	no	Murata et al. 1999
Pruritic eruption of pregnancy	PCR	skin	yes	Aractingi et al. 1998

Table 3. Maternal cells in human diseases

Disease	Detection technique	Sample	Increase in cell number	Reference(s)
Systemic sclerosis	HLA-specific PCR and FISH	blood	no	Maloney et al. 1999
Myositis	PCR, FISH	blood, tissue	yes	Reed et al. 2000, Artlett et al. 2000
GVHD in immuno-deficiency	HLA typing	blood	no controls	Wirt et al. 1982, Pollack et al. 1982

contribute to her immune tolerance of the fetus, which is effectively an allograft that would be expected to be rejected.

Since microchimerism is a common event, if such foreign cells are involved in autoimmune disease, then there must be additional factors triggering the cells to persistently induce inflammation. Further studies are needed to determine whether microchimerism contributes to disease pathogenesis in the context of other factors such as environmental or infectious triggers and HLA relationships of host and nonhost cells. Maternal-fetal compatibility has been associated with the development of SSc, and in particular HLA alleles have been associated with increased frequency of microchimerism. If fetal and/or maternal microchimerism are found to be involved in the pathogenesis of autoimmune disease, then a whole new class of therapeutic agents may be developed to target these foreign cells.

References

Aractingi S, Berkane N, Bertheau P, et al (1998) Fetal DNA in skin of polymorphic eruptions of pregnancy. Lancet 352: 1898–1901

Arnett FC, Howard RF, Tan F, et al (1996) Increased prevalence of systemic sclerosis in a Native American tribe in Oklahoma: association with an Amerindian HLA haplotype. Arthritis Rheum 39: 1362–1370

Artlett CM, Welsh KI, Black CM, Jimenez SA (1997) Fetal-maternal HLA compatibility confers suscepti-bility to systemic sclerosis. Immunogenetics 47: 17–22

Artlett CM, Smith JB, Jimenez SA (1998) Identification of fetal DNA and cells in skin lesions from women with systemic sclerosis. N Engl J Med 338: 1186–1191

Artlett CM, Ramos R, Jiminez SA, Patterson K, Miller FW, Rider LG (2000a) Chimeric cells of maternal origin in juvenile idiopathic inflammatory myopathies. Lancet 356: 2155–2156

Artlett CM, Cox LA, Jimenez SA (2000b) Detection of cellular microchimerism of male or female origin in systemic sclerosis patients by polymerase chain reaction analysis of HLA-Cw antigens. Arthritis Rheum 43: 1062–1067

Bianchi DW, Zickwolf GK, Weil GJ, Sylvester S, DeMaria MA (1996) Male fetal progenitor cells persist in maternal blood for as long as 27 years postpartum. Proc Natl Acad Sci USA 93: 705–708

Bianchi DW, Farina A, Weber W, et al (2001) Significant fetal-maternal hemorrhage after termination of pregnancy: implications for development of fetal cell microchimerism. Am J Obstet Gynecol 184: 703–706

Christner PJ, Artlett CM, Conway RF, Jimenez SA (2000) Increased numbers of microchimeric cells of fetal origin are associated with dermal fibrosis in mice following injection of vinyl chloride. Arthritis Rheum 43: 2598–2605

Corpechot C, Barbu V, Chazouilleres O, Poupon R (2000) Fetal microchimerism in primary biliary cirrhosis. J Hepatol 33: 696–700

De Moor G, De Bock G, Noens L, De Bie S (1988) A new case of human chimerism detected after preg-nancy: 46,XY karyotype in the lymphocytes of a woman. Acta Clin Belg 43: 231–235

Evans PC, Lambert N, Maloney S, Furst DE, Moore JM, Nelson JL (1999) Long-term fetal microchimerism in peripheral blood mononuclear cell subsets in healthy women and women with scleroderma. Blood 93: 2033–2037

Fanning PA, Jonsson JR, Clouston AD, et al (2000) Detection of male DNA in the liver of female patients with primary biliary cirrhosis. J Hepatol 33: 690–695

Gelpi C, Martinez MA, Vidal S, Targoff IN, Rodriguez-Sanchez JL (1994) Autoantibodies to a transfer RNA-associated protein in a murine model of chronic graft versus host disease. J Immunol 152: 1989–1999

Gleichmann E, Van Elven EH, Van der Veen JP (1982) A systemic lupus erythematosus (SLE)-like disease in mice induced by abnormal T-B cell cooperation: preferential formation of autoantibodies characteristic of SLE. Eur J Immunol 12: 152–159

Hall JM, Lingenfelter P, Adams SL, Lasser D, Hansen JA, Bean MA (1995) Detection of maternal cells in human umbilical cord blood using fluorescence in situ hybridization. Blood 86: 2829–2832

Ichikawa N, Kotake S, Hakoda M, Kamatani N (2001) Microchimerism in Japanese patients with systemic sclerosis. Arthritis Rheum 44: 1226–1228

Invernizzi P, De Andreis C, Sirchia SM, et al (2000) Blood fetal microchimerism in primary biliary cirrhosis. Clin Exp Immunol 122: 418–422

Johnson KL, Nelson JL, Furst DE, et al (2001) Fetal cell microchimerism in tissue from multiple sites in women with systemic sclerosis. Arthritis Rheum 44: 1848–1854

Klintschar M, Schwaiger P, Mannweiler S, Regauer S, Kleiber M (2001) Evidence of fetal microchimerism in Hashimoto's thyroiditis. J Clin Endocrinol Metab 86: 2494–2498

Lambe M, Hsieh C, Trichopoulos D, Ekbom A, Pavia M, Adami HO (1994) Transient increase in the risk of breast cancer after giving birth. N Engl J Med 331: 5–9

Lambert NC, Distler O, Muller-Ladner U, Tylee TS, Furst DE, Nelson JL (2000a) HLA-DQA1*0501 is associated with diffuse systemic sclerosis in Caucasian men. Arthritis Rheum 43: 2005–2010

Lambert NC, Evans PC, Hashizumi TL, et al (2000b) Cutting edge: persistent fetal microchimerism in T lymphocytes is associated with HLA-DQA1*0501: implications in autoimmunity. J Immunol 164: 5545–5548

Lee TH, Paglieroni T, Ohto H, Holland PV, Busch MP (1999) Survival of donor leukocyte subpopulations in immunocompetent transfusion recipients: frequent long-term microchimerism in severe trauma patients. Blood 93: 3127–3139

Lo YM, Lo ES, Watson N, et al (1996) Two-way cell traffic between mother and fetus: biologic and clinical implications. Blood 88: 4390–4395

Lo YM, Lau TK, Chan LY, Leung TN, Chang AM (2000) Quantitative analysis of the bidirectional fetomaternal transfer of nucleated cells and plasma DNA. Clin Chem 46: 1301–1309

Maloney S, Smith A, Furst DE, et al (1999) Microchimerism of maternal origin persists into adult life. J Clin Invest 104: 41–47

McMilin KD, Johnson RL (1993) HLA homozygosity and the risk of related-donor transfusion-associated graft-versus-host disease. Transfus Med Rev 7: 37–41

Miyashita Y, Ono M, Ueki H, Kurasawa K (2000) Y chromosome microchimerism in rheumatic autoimmune disease. Ann Rheum Dis 59: 655–656

Morrow J, Nelson J, Watts R, Isenberg D (1999) Autoimmune rheumatic disease. Oxford University Press, Oxford

Mullinax F (1993) Chimerism and autoimmunity. In: Proceedings of the Fourth ASEAN Congress of Rheumatology, Singapore, October 31 to November 4, 1993, pp 39–40

Murata H, Nakauchi H, Sumida T (1999) Microchimerism in Japanese women patients with systemic sclerosis. Lancet 354: 220–00

Nelson JL, Hughes KA, Smith AG, Nisperos BB, Branchaud AM, Hansen JA (1993) Maternal-fetal disparity in HLA class II alloantigens and the pregnancy-induced amelioration of rheumatoid arthritis. N Engl J Med 329: 466–471

Nelson JL, Furst DE, Maloney S, et al (1998) Microchimerism and HLA-compatible relationships of pregnancy in scleroderma. Lancet 351: 559–562

Nelson JL (1996) Maternal-fetal immunology and autoimmune disease: is some autoimmune disease auto-alloimmune or allo-autoimmune? Arthritis Rheum 39: 191–194

Petit T, Gluckman E, Carosella E, Brossard Y, Brison O, Socie G (1995) A highly sensitive polymerase chain reaction method reveals the ubiquitous presence of maternal cells in human umbilical cord blood. Exp Hematol 23: 1601–1605

Petit T, Dommergues M, Socie G, Dumez Y, Gluckman E, Brison O (1997) Detection of maternal cells in human fetal blood during the third trimester of pregnancy using allele-specific PCR amplification. Br J Haematol 98: 767–771

Pollack MS, Kirkpatrick D, Kapoor N, Dupont B, O'Reilly RJ (1982) Identification by HLA typing of intrauterine-derived maternal T cells in four patients with severe combined immunodeficiency. N Engl J Med 307: 662–666

Portanova JP, Ebling FM, Hammond WS, Hahn BH, Kotzin BL (1988) Allogeneic MHC antigen requirements for lupus-like autoantibody production and nephritis in murine graft-vs-host disease. J Immunol 141: 3370–3376

Reed A, Picnorell YJ, Harwood A, Kredich D (2000) Chimerism in children with juvenile dermatomyositis. Lancet 356: 2156–2157

Rouquette-Gally AM, Boyeldieu D, Gluckman E, Abuaf N, Combrisson A (1987) Autoimmunity in 28 patients after allogeneic bone marrow transplantation: comparison with Sjogren syndrome and scleroderma. Br J Haematol 66: 45–47

Rubbia-Brandt L, Philippeaux MM, Chavez S, Mentha G, Borisch B, Hadengue A (1999) FISH for Y chromosome in women with primary biliary cirrhosis: lack of evidence for leukocyte microchimerism. Hepatology 30: 821–822

Srivatsa B, Srivatsa S, Johnson KL, Samura O, Lee SL, Bianchi DW (2001) Microchimerism of presumed fetal origin in thyroid specimens from women: a case-control study. Lancet 358: 2034–2038

Stevens AM, Hermes H, Nelson JL (2001a) Maternal microchimerism in neonatal lupus erythematosus (NLE) [abstract]. Arthritis Rheum 44: S160

Stevens AM, Hermes H, Tylee T, Nelson JL (2001b) Maternal microchimerism in the human thymus [abstract]. Arthritis Rheum 44: S340

Tanaka A, Lindor K, Ansari A, Gershwin ME (2000) Fetal microchimerisms in the mother: immunologic implications. Liver Transpl 6: 138–143

Thomas MR, Williamson R, Craft I, Yazdani N, Rodeck CH (1994) Y chromosome sequence DNA ampli-
    fied from peripheral blood of women in early pregnancy [letter]. Lancet 343: 413–414
Toda I, Kuwana M, Tsubota K, Kawakami Y (2001) Lack of evidence for an increased microchimerism in
    the circulation of patients with Sjogren's syndrome. Ann Rheum Dis 60: 248–253
Vietor HE (1998) Immunomodulation induced by intrauterine transfusions. Eur J Obstet Gynecol Reprod
    Biol 78: 33–35
Vietor HE, Hamel BC, van Bree SP, et al (2000) Immunological tolerance in an HLA non-identical
    chimeric twin. Hum Immunol 61: 190–192
Wirt DP, Brooks EG, Vaidya S, Klimpel GR, Waldmann TA, Goldblum RM (1989) Novel T-lymphocyte
    population in combined immunodeficiency with features of graft-versus-host disease. N Engl J Med 321:
    370–374

Therapeutic aspects of autoimmune diseases of the skin

Michael Sticherling*

Department of Dermatology, University of Leipzig, Leipzig, Federal Republic of Germany

Introduction

The skin represents the largest and at the same time most exposed organ of the human body. Apart from infectious, inflammatory, and neoplastic conditions it can be involved by autoimmune reactions as well. These may result in distinct clinical entities where the skin is the main or only target as found among autoimmune bullous skin diseases. In contrast, skin symptoms are seen as one of several disease manifestations in the context of collagenoses which represent multiorgan diseases. A third group of skin manifestations presents with uncharacteristic symptoms which simply reflect autoimmune diseases of internal organs (Table 1).

The impact of both basic and clinical immunology has changed the attitudes towards pathogenesis and therapeutic approaches of autoimmune disorders. Within these, skin autoimmune diseases may serve as model diseases for other organs (Robert and Kupper 1999, Krueger 2002). Especially the progress in transplantation medicine has grossly enlarged the therapeutic armentarium (Table 2). In dermatology, the affected organ is easily accessible from outside. Therefore both the local, external and the systemic, internal treatment are effective and well established. Similar to other organs, skin autoimmune diseases are induced by either

Table 1. Autoimmune diseases of the skin

Primary autoimmune disease	Skin as only target organ with characteristic symptoms
Secondary autoimmune disease	Skin as one of several target organs with characteristic symptoms
Symptomatic disease	Skin organ mirroring internal disease with uncharacteristic symptoms
Hypothetic/possible autoimmune disease	Skin disease with possible autoimmune background

* Author's address: Department of Dermatology, University of Leipzig, Stephanstrasse 9, 04103 Leipzig, Federal Republic of Germany.
E-mail: sticm@medizin.uni-leipzig.de

Table 2. Therapeutic options

Established	Experimental	Future
corticosteroids	IVIG	monoclonal antibodies
azathioprine	MMF	fusion proteins
methotrexate	leflunomide	antisense oligonucleotides
cyclophosphamide	plasmapheresis	peptide vaccination
cyclosporin	photopheresis	
cytokines	monoclonal antibodies	
antibiotics	fusion proteins	
dapsone	thalidomide	

cellular, mostly T-cell-mediated, or humoral reactions. Their relative involvement in the pathogenesis of individual diseases is not known in many cases. Consequently, therapeutic approaches have often been based on anecdotal application and empirical knowledge rather than on evidence-based studies and pathogenic knowledge. On the other side, the effectiveness of some well-established, traditional therapeutic strategies can now be explained by recent advances of immunology (Table 2).

Autoimmune diseases of the skin

Primary autoimmune diseases of the skin

These diseases present with manifestations restricted to the skin and mucous membranes. Further symptoms are only secondary to complications like infection and dysbalance of electrolyte and water (Table 1). Classical diseases within this group encompass autoimmune bullous skin diseases. In most of these, specific humoral, antibody-mediated mechanisms result in a disruption of cell contact within the epidermis or between epidermis and dermis. Detection of antibodies locally deposited at these sites as well as circulating specific antibodies within the blood are now widely used for diagnostic purposes. The progress of molecular biology has helped to characterize the various antigens involved. Thus distinct disease subgroups can be further dissected which results in improved disease nomenclature. On the basis of this heterogeneity in regard to humoral as well as cellular causes, the clinical experience of varying therapeutic responses and prognoses of apparently similar or homogeneous diseases may now be explained. Until today, glucocorticoids present the mainstay of therapeutic intervention. In fact, before their availability diseases like bullous pemphigoid (BP) and even more pemphigus (PV) presented with an excessive short-term mortality of 60–100%. Usually these diseases require sustained immunosuppressive treatment with initially high doses of corticosteroids for rapid clinical effects in addition to adjuvant drugs with delayed but steroid-sparing effects.

Within this group of diseases, dermatitis herpetiformis Duhring may be regarded as an own entity or skin manifestation of celiac disease. Distinct differences among these diseases regarding incidence, age of onset, gender predisposition, rate of coincidence, and therapeutic response indicate distinct but related diseases.

Secondary autoimmune diseases of the skin

Within this disease group, the skin represents one of several targets with characteristic clinical symptoms. This applies to the different entities among the collagenous disorders. These may present with skin symptoms either as initial manifestation or later during the course of disease as seen in lupus erythematosus, systemic scleroderma, and dermatomyositis. All three denominations refer to characteristic skin symptoms within these diseases. In any of them, Raynaud phenomenon, livedo-like skin pattern and nail-fold abnormalities can be found. Skin symptoms of lupus erythematosus (LE) are differently appreciated in dermatology and rheumatology as either only symptomatic or own entities. Whereas chronic cutaneous LE and subacute cutaneous LE show well-defined skin lesions, systemic LE may present with any of these or other less characteristic symptoms like rashes, urticaria or skin vasculitis or may even miss any major skin involvement. Regarding this overlap, every cutaneous LE patient has to be carefully evaluated to exclude incipient systemic disease. Regarding therapeutic approaches, pulmonary, cardial, and renal involvement mainly dictate the prognosis of the disease. However, in many cases internal organ involvement can be properly handled at drug doses where skin symptoms will still be present and result in gross distress. In addition to collagenoses, other rheumatoid diseases and different forms of primary systemic vasculitis may present with more or less characteristic skin symptoms like purpura, inflammatory papules, erosions, and ulcerations as well as rashes. As patients often present initially with skin symptoms, a careful case history of other constitutive signs may give indication of underlying systemic disease and results in adequate diagnostic measures.

Symptomatic skin involvement in autoimmune diseases

In these diseases, the skin is indirectly involved. As the most exposed human organ, it may just mirror internal disease with uncharacteristic symptoms. These include skin dryness in thyroid disease, intense pruritus and resulting eczematous reactions in renal disease, jaundice in hepatic disorders, or secondary involvement through long-term complications of underlying autoimmune diseases. In diabetes mellitus, peripheral gangrene and acral ulcerations can be found as a result of peripheral neuropathy or disrupted arterial circulation. Therapy of skin manifestations will be symptomatic and only successful if the underlying disease is properly treated at the same time.

Hypothetic/possible autoimmune disease

During the last decades following expanding immunological knowledge, many skin diseases have been pathogenetically defined by perturbed immunological responses to exogenous damage, especially infectious agents. Even if autoimmune phenomena are involved, their relevance among pathogenic mechanisms has still to be evaluated in detail. In this respect, psoriasis as one of the most common chronic inflammatory skin diseases is much speculated upon. Apart from suspected parainfectious immunological reactions, underlying metabolic disorders and a genetic predisposition towards chronic skin inflammatory reactions, autoimmune phenomena have been found directed towards epidermal, possibly keratinocyte antigens.

Therapeutic concepts for skin autoimmune diseases

Therapeutic interventions have to be differentially introduced depending on the kind of dermatological disease, the extent of organ involvement other than skin as well as the degree of inflammatory activity (Table 2). This determines the decision for external or internal treatment, its dosage and duration. In multiorgan autoimmune diseases, skin involvement usually does neither indicate disease activity nor pose a live-threatening manifestation. However, dermal manifestations may be badly disabling or cosmetically disturbing and result in a distinct reduction of quality of live.

On the basis of these concepts, current dermatological therapeutic strategies for autoimmune diseases include cytotoxic, immunosuppressive, and immunomodulatory drugs and are further discussed in the following sections (Dutz and Ho 1998, Luger 2001, Thoma-Uszynski and Hertl 2001, Sticherling 2001, Sapadin and Fleischmajer 2002, Krueger 2002).

Local immunomodulatory treatment

As the most exposed organ of the human body, the skin is easily accessible from outside. However, many immunosuppressive drugs are not available for local treatment or do not penetrate the horny layer in sufficient amounts to reach both the vital epidermis and the dermal compartment. Thus, effective local treatment is mainly restricted to corticosteroids. They are available at different pharmacological strengths regarding anti-inflammatory activity as well as local side effects. These include induction of skin atrophy, acneiform disease, teleangiectasia as well as hyper- and hypopigmentation. In addition, the local immune response is suppressed to result in an increased incidence of skin infections. Corticosteroids are available in different ointment confections for external application, adhesive crèmes or solutions for mucus membranes or for local intra- and sublesional injection. Local or restricted manifestation of bullous pemphigoid as well as cutaneous manifestations of LE can be successfully treated with local corticosteroids (Glied and Rico 1999, Joly et al. 2002). In many cases however, especially with extensive skin involvement, systemic treatment is necessary. Additional local antiseptic treatment is mandatory to prevent bacterial or fungal skin infections.

Interesting novel immunomodulatory substances are about to be introduced into dermatology for local treatment like macrolactames (Bornhovd et al. 2001, Thoma-Uszynski and Hertl 2001). As they have been derived from systemic treatment, they will be discussed below. Vitamin D derivatives represent another interesting group of components which is well established in dermatology for the local treatment of psoriasis and is increasingly used for skin autoimmune diseases (Ameen et al. 2001, Ermis et al. 2001, Lamba and Lebwohl 2001). Apart from antiproliferative effects as well as induction of differentiation in epidermal keratinocytes, inhibition of adhesion molecules and lymphocyte functions indicate immunomodulatory activity of these compounds. In case reports as well as initial studies, they have successfully been used in alopecia areata, vitiligo, and localized scleroderma/morphea. In addition to local use, systemic vitamin D derivatives may in the future be used for immunomodulation, though the components available so far show distinct and limiting side effects on calcium and phosphate balance. Similarly, the use of systemic vitamin A derivatives is well established in dermatology including cutaneous LE (Sticherling 2001). Local treatment has become available recently (tazarotene) and may be used in chronic discoid LE (Edwards and Burke 1999).

A novel immunomodulatory substance, imiquimod, has been recently introduced and licensed for use in human papillomavirus infections of the skin and mucous membranes (Sauder 2000). Its effects are mediated by local induction of alpha and gamma interferon and interleukin-12 and -8. The activation of macrophages, T cells, and natural killer cells will induce effective local immune response. Apart from papillomavirus clearance, clinical effectiveness has been shown for epithelial skin tumours like squamous cell carcinoma and basal cell carcinoma. On the basis of these results, the local application of imiquimod in skin autoimmune diseases like alopecia areata and cutaneous LE is currently evaluated.

Another local, that is, external treatment modality almost exclusively used in dermatology is ultraviolet light (Gasparro 2000). The differential immunomodulatory activity of both UV-A (alone or in combination with UV-sensitizing drugs) and UV-B is well appreciated regarding Langerhans cell and lymphocyte activity. UV therapy is therapeutically used for psoriasis, atopic eczema, lichen ruber to list a few. Therapeutic effectiveness is however restricted and has been described for PUVA treatment of systemic scleroderma or UV-A1 treatment of LE.

Systemic immunomodulatory drugs

Immunosuppression is classically achieved by glucocorticosteroids and cytotoxic drugs like cyclophosphamide (Fleischli et al. 1999). Established strategies are supplemented by alternative, second- or third-line as well as experimental approaches. Systemic corticosteroids are widely and effectively used in skin autoimmune diseases (Werth 1993, Becker et al. 1998). Their importance in first-line treatment of autoimmune disorders has not been diminished by the availability of modern immunomodulatory drugs as their clinical effects are much more rapid and effective in the initial phase of disease. Regarding distinct short- and long-term side effects of corticosteroids in chronic diseases, they need to be tapered and combined with other immunosuppressive drugs with delayed onset of effects (see below). Accordingly, the reluctance of both medical doctors and patients to use corticosteroids has to be balanced by their effectiveness, resulting in critical and responsible use. Laboratory examination as well as bone densitometry have to be performed before initiation of steroid therapy as well as in regular intervals during treatment. Recommendations for such examinations and their consequences on initiation of corticosteroids have only recently been given (Genant et al. 1999). The doses and durations of therapy are varying to a great extent among the different dermatologically relevant autoimmune diseases (listed in Tables 1 and 2). These clinical regimens have been established empirically over many years and decades, most of them have, however, not been evaluated in clinical studies fulfilling the criteria for evidence-based medicine nor regarding the recent diagnostic advances in many of these diseases. Even more, these traditional regimens are used as gold standard in studies evaluating novel immunomodulatory drugs. This problem is reflected within the therapy of bullous pemphigoid, which mostly affects patients well above the age of 60 with increased risk of drug-induced side effects (Glied and Rico 1999). The initial dose of corticosteroids is still set at 1 mg/kg of body weight or above in a disease which might often be equally well treated by alternative drugs with distinctly lower side effects. Adequate clinical studies are needed and will be initiated soon (Joly et al. 2002, Rzany et al. 2002).

Adjuvant drugs

Corticosteroids are usually combined with other immunomodulatory drugs which allow tapering of steroid dose or show additive or supportive effects. They may be used as monotherapy in mild disease or after stopping steroids. Often these are called adjuvant drugs. Azathioprine is most often used in this context at a dose of 1–2 mg/kg of body weight. Thiopurine methyltransferase activity should be evaluated before initiating the therapy to lower the incidence of side effects (Anstey 1996, Tan et al. 1997). These mainly consist of disturbed blood count, apart from alopecia, arthralgia and skin as well as neoplasia in the long run. Alternatively, methotrexate may be used both in autoimmune bullous skin disease (BP, PV) as well as collagenous diseases (LE, dermatomyositis) apart from psoriasis (Bottomley and Goodfield 1995, Mrowietz 2001). Doses at 15–25 mg once per week are very effective and can be given intravenously or orally. As with azathioprine, blood count and liver enzymes should be regularly checked (Cronstein 1996, Jeffes et al. 1995).

Both chloroquin and hydroxychloroquin are used as basic adjuvant drug for the treatment of rheumatic disorders and were shown to be effective in skin manifestations of LE (Sticherling 2001, Ochsendorf and Runne 1996).

As an alternative adjuvant drug thalidomide has been reintroduced into clinical use in other diseases than lepra, especially for treatment of refractory cutaneous LE. On the basis of the modulation of tumor necrosis factor alpha (TNF-α) release, chronic inflammatory skin diseases, especially those with granuloma formation, are successfully treated (Georgala et al. 1998, Warren et al. 1998, Kyriakis et al. 2000, Ordi-Ros et al. 2000). In autoimmune bullous skin disease, especially bullous pemphigoid, diaminodiphenylsulfone (dapsone), tetracycline antibiotics and nicotinamide as well as colchizine can be very effectively used alone or in combination with corticosteroids. They help to circumvent steroid-induced side effects in elderly patients. The clinical effectiveness of dapsone could recently be explained by demonstrating in vitro the inhibition of interleukin-8 and TNF-α

release as well as of chemotactic migration of neutrophilic granulocytes (Wozel 1996). This is an example for other drugs which have been known to be clinically effective for a long time. With current advances in immunological knowledge, their mode of action can now be explained.

Another treatment modality with adjuvant effect is represented by intravenous immunoglobulins. These polyclonal-antibody preparations from pool sera of selected donors are licenced for primary and secondary immunodeficiency as well as Kawasaki syndrome and idiopathic thrombopenic purpura. Their effectiveness in dermatomyositis is well documented in several case reports as well as blinded studies (Dalakas 1999). Furthermore, different autoimmune bullous skin diseases like pemphigus vulgaris and bullous pemphigoid have been treated successfully apart from LE (Ahmed 2001, Bodemer et al. 1990, De Vita et al. 1996, Jolles et al. 1998, O'Donnell et al. 1998, Roujeau 1999, Rabinovitch et al. 1999, Sacher 2001, Sadayama et al. 1999). They have been used at doses from 0.1 to 2 g/kg of body weight. Both humoral and cellular specific and nonspecific mechanisms have been described to explain therapeutic responses. Regarding the pathogenetically very heterogeneic autoimmune diseases, different mechanisms of action seem effective. There is consent that in these diseases intravenous immunoglobulins should be used when standard therapy regimens have failed and in combination only (Sacher 2001). The high costs of each single cycle have to be balanced against all other costs deriving from the debilitating and chronic diseases.

Other adjuvant drugs with immunomodulatory activity have been developed and licensed for use in transplantation medicine and introduced into dermatology to treat immunologically mediated skin disorders (Dutz and Ho 1998, Luger 2001, Mrowietz 2000, Thoma-Uszynski and Hertl 2001). Their main target are lymphocytes which are modulated in respect to their proliferation and functional activities, e.g., in respect to cytokine production. These drugs include mycophenolate mofetil (Jayne 1999, Furst 1999) and leflunomide (Kurtz et al. 1995, Parnham 1995, Furst 1999, Glant et al. 1998, Nousari and Anhalt 2000) as purin and pyrimidine antagonists respectively on the one hand and cyclosporin A (Saeki et al. 2000) as well as macrolide antibiotics like FK506 (tacrolimus), ascomycin (pimecrolimus), and rapamycin (sirolimus) (Bornhovd et al. 2001, Luger 2001, Thoma-Uszynski and Hertl 2001) on the other hand, which are mainly involved in the calmodulin-calcineurin-mediated signal transmission pathways. Thus the expression of both Th1 and Th2 cytokines is inhibited, resulting in a modulation of T cell responses. Apart from cyclosporin A for psoriasis none is licensed yet for use in dermatology, though tacrolimus will follow soon for atopic dermatitis. However, the number of case reports on the use of any of these drugs in a variety of dermatological autoimmune diseases is steadily increasing but still has to be evaluated in clinical studies. In a recent German multicenter study the effects of a combination of systemic corticosteroids with either mycophenolate mofetil or azathioprine have been compared in autoimmune bullous skin disease and results will be available soon. The same applies to the clinical effectiveness of tacrolimus and ascomycin, which apart from systemic use are available for local application.

Fumaric acid derivatives repesent systemically active agents which have been exclusively used in dermatology for a long time. Their effects on keratinocyte and lymphocyte functions as well as their clinical effectiveness are well documented (Altmeyer et al. 1994, Mrowietz et al. 1999). They have however been hardly used for the treatment of other diseases than psoriasis. Their mode of action as well as the accumulating experience suggests that they may be applicable in autoimmune disorders as well.

Other immunologically based therapeutic approaches

Apart from local and systemic treatment options as outlined above, a number of extracorporeal approaches have been applied in dermatology (Thoma-Uszynski and Hertl 2001). In B-cell-antibody-mediated skin autoimmune diseases, the pathogenetically relevant autoantibodies can either be separated nonselectively together with other plasma proteins as in plasmapheresis or semiselectively together with other immunoglobulins as in immunoabsorption. The progress in characterizing the relevant target autoantigens as well as their availability as recombinant proteins will soon result in affinity columns selectively separating specific antibodies. Extracorporeal photophoresis (Richter et al. 1998, Wollina and Looks 1999) represents another approach targeting mainly T cells and macrophages and has successfully been used for systemic scleroderma as well as LE.

Future and experimental therapeutic approaches

Cytokines, mainly interleukin-2 and interferons, have been used for diverse autoimmune diseases including those of the skin (Thivolet et al. 1990, Luger 2001). Major studies have been performed on systemic scleroderma and LE (Sapadin and Fleischmajer 2002). The availability of monoclonal antibodies as well as fusion proteins for therapeutic purposes has dramatically increased over the last years (Prinz et al. 1996, Gelfand 2001, Luger 2001, Isaacs 2001). Their effectiveness in dermatological autoimmune diseases is well documented. The various immunologically relevant target antigens include surface proteins like adhesion molecules, lymphocyte receptors, and cytokines as well as their receptors. Another approach is immunoablative treatment of severe skin autoimmune diseases followed by bone marrow stem cell transplantation (Burt et al. 2002). Other approaches like antisense oligonucleotides to cytokines and lymphocyte activation proteins as well as peptide vaccination to specifically prevent or reverse immunological sensitization are still in the experimental stage.

Outlook

The concept of dermatological diseases has dramatically changed following the progress of basic and clinical immunology over recent years. Many skin diseases which have remained unexplained for a long time were shown to be immunologically mediated, many of them with distinct autoimmune phenomena. Following this concept, therapeutic approaches are targeting this disturbed immunological balance. Apart from local treatment, systemic immunomodulatory regimens derived from transplantation medicine are introduced into dermatology. At the same time many immunologically mediated skin diseases with distinct autoimmune phenomena like psoriasis may serve as models for other inflammatory diseases. Both clinical effectiveness and side effects of novel therapeutic approaches can be monitored at the skin organ, which is immunologically competent and at the same time easily accessible. Accordingly, novel therapeutic approaches derived from other organs can be transferred to dermatology as vice versa the experience from the treatment of dermatological diseases can be transferred to autoimmune diseases of other organs.

References

Ahmed AR (2001) Intravenous immunoglobulin therapy for patients with bullous pemphigoid unresponsive to conventional immunosuppressive treatment. J Am Acad Dermatol 45: 825–835

Altmeyer P, Matthes U, Pawlak F, Hoffmann K, Frosch PJ, Ruppert P (1994) Antipsoriatic effect of fumaric acid derivatives: results of a multicenter double-blind study in 100 patients. J Am Acad Dermatol 30: 977–981

Ameen M, Exarchou V, Chu AC (2001) Topical calcipotriol as monotherapy and in combination with psoralen plus ultraviolet A in the treatment of vitiligo. Br J Dermatol 145: 476–479

Anstey A (1996) Management of immunobullous disorders: the clinical significance of interindividual variation in azathioprine metabolism. Clin Exp Dermatol 21: 247–248

Becker L, Bastian B, Wesselmann U, Karl S, Hamm H, Bröcker EB (1998) Paraneoplastic pemphigus treated with dexamethasone/cyclophosphamide pulse therapy. Eur J Dermatol 8: 551–553

Bodemer C, Teillac D, Le Bourgeois M, Wechsler B, de Prost Y (1990) Efficacy of intravenous immunglobulins in sclerodermatomyositis. Br J Dermatol 123: 545–546

Bornhovd E, Burgdorf WH, Wollenberg A (2001) Macrolactam immunomodulators for topical treatment of inflammatory skin diseases. J Am Acad Dermatol 45: 736–743

Bottomley WW, Goodfield MJ (1995) Methotrexate for the treatment of discoid lupus erythematosus. Br J Dermatol 133: 655–656

Burt RK, Slavin S, Burns WH, Marmont AM (2002) Induction of tolerance in autoimmune diseases by hematopoietic stem cell transplantation: getting closer to a cure? Blood 99: 768–784

Cronstein BN (1996) Molecular therapeutics: methotrexate and its mechanism of action. Arthritis Rheum 39: 1951–1960

Dalakas MC (1999) Intravenous immunoglobulin in the treatment of autoimmune neuromuscular diseases: present status and practical therapeutic guidelines. Muscle Nerve 22: 1479–1497

De Vita S, Ferraccioli GF, Di Poi E, Bartoli E, Bombardieri S (1996) High dose intravenous immunoglobulin therapy for rheumatic diseases: clinical relevance and personal experience. Clin Exp Rheumatol 14: S85–S92

Dutz JP, Ho VC (1998) Immunosuppressive agents in dermatology: an update. Dermatol Clin 16: 235–251

Edwards KR, Burke WA (1999) Treatment of localized discoid lupus erythematosus with tazarotene. J Am Acad Dermatol 41: 1049–1050

Ermis O, Alpsoy LC, Yilmaz E (2001) Is the efficacy of psoralen plus ultraviolet A therapy for vitiligo enhanced by concurrent topical calcipotriol? A placebo-controlled double-blind study. Br J Dermatol 145: 472–475

Fleischli ME, Rachel H, Valek BS, Pandya AG (1999) Pulse intravenous cyclophosphamide therapy in pemphigus. Arch Dermatol 135: 57–61

Furst DE (1999) Leflunomide, mycophenolic acid and matrix metalloproteinase inhibitors. Rheumatology (Oxford) 38: 14–18

Gasparro FP (2000) Photodermatology: progress, problems and prospects. Eur J Dermatol 10: 250–254

Gelfand Erwin W (2001) Antibody-directed therapy: past, present and future. J Allergy Clin Immunol 108: 111–116

Genant HK, Cooper C, Poor G, Reid I, Ehrlich G, Kanis J, Nordin BE, Barrett-Connor E, Black D, Bonjour JP, Dawson-Hughes B, Delmas PD, Dequeker J, Ragi Eis S, Gennari C, Johnell O, Johnston CC Jr, Lau EM, Liberman UA, Lindsay R, Martin TJ, Masri B, Mautalen CA, Meunier PJ, Khaltaev N (1999)

Interim report and recommendations of the World Health Organization Task-Force for Osteoporosis. Osteoporos Int 10: 259–264

Georgala S, Katoulis AC, Hasapi V, Koumantaki-Mathioudaki E (1998) Thalidomide treatment for hypertrophic lupus erythematosus. Clin Exp Dermatol 23: 141

Glant TT, Mikecz K, Brennan F, Negroiu G, Bartlett R (1998) Suppression of autoimmune responses and inflammatory events by leflunomide in an animal model for rheumatoid arthritis. J Rheumatol 25: 20–26

Glied M, Rico MJ (1999) Treatment of autoimmune blistering diseases. Dermatol Clin 17: 431–440

Isaacs JD (2001) From bench to bedside: discovering rules for antibody design, and improving serotherapy with monclonal antibodies. Rheumatology (Oxford) 40: 724–738

Jayne D (1999) Non-transplant uses of mycophenolate mofetil. Curr Opin Nephrol Hypertens 8: 563–567

Jeffes EW 3rd, McCullough JL, Pittelkow MR, McCormick A, Almanzor J, Liu G, et al (1995) Methotrexate therapy of psoriasis: differential sensitivity of proliferating lymphoid and epithelial cells to the cytotoxic and growth–inhibitory effects of methotrexate. J Invest Dermatol 104: 184–188

Jolles S, Hughes J, Whittaker S (1998) Dermatological uses of high-dose intravenous immunoglobulin. Arch Dermatol 134: 80–86

Joly P, Roujeau JC, Benichou J, Picard C, Dreno B, Delaporte E, Vaillant L, D'Incan M, Plantin P, Bedane C, Young P, Bernard P, The Bullous Diseases French Study Group (2002) A comparison of oral and topical corticosteroids in patients with bullous pemphigoid. N Engl J Med 346: 321–327

Krueger JG (2002) The immunologic basis for the treatment of psoriasis with new biologic agents. J Am Acad Dermatol 46: 1–23

Kurtz ES, Bayley SC, Arshad F, Lee AA, Przekop PA (1995) Leflunomide: an active antiinflammatory and antiproliferative agent in models of dermatologic disease. Inflamm Res 44: 187–188

Kyriakis KP, Kontochristopoulos GJ, Panteleos DN (2000) Experience with low-dose thalidomide therapy in chronic discoid lupus erythematosus. Int J Dermatol 39: 218–222

Lamba S, Lebwohl M (2001) Combination therapy with vitamin D analogues. Br J Dermatol 144: 27–32

Luger T (2001) Treatment of immune-mediated skin diseases: future perspectives. Eur J Dermatol 11: 343–347

Mrowietz U (2001) Advances in systemic therapy for psoriasis. Clin Dermatol 26: 362–367

Mrowietz U, Christophers E, Altmeyer P (1999) Treamtent of severe psoriasis with fumaric acid esters: scientific background and guidelines for therapeutic use. Br J Dermatol 141: 424–429

Nousari HG, Anhalt GJ (2000) Bullous pemphigoid treated with leflunomide. Arch Dermatol 136: 1204–1205

Ochsendorf FR, Runne U (1996) Chloroquine: consideration of maximum daily dose (3.5 mg/kg ideal body weigth) prevents retinopathy. Dermatology 192: 382–383

O'Donnell BF, Barr RM, Black AK, Francis DM, Kermani F, Niimi N, Barlow RJ, Winkelmann RK, Greaves MW (1998) Intravenous immunoglobulin in autoimmune chronic urticaria. Br J Dermatol 138: 101–106

Ordi-Ros J, Cortes F, Cucrull E, Mauri M, Bujan S, Vilardell M (2000) Thalidomide in the treatment of cutaneous lupus refractory to conventional therapy. J Rheumatol 27: 1429–1433

Parnham MJ (1995) Leflunomide: a potential new disease modifying anti-rheumatic drug. Exp Opin Invest Drugs 4: 777–779

Prinz JC, Meurer M, Reiter C, Rieber EP, Plewig G, Riethmuller G (1996) Treatment of severe cutaneous lupus erythematosus with a chimeric CD4 monoclonal antibody, cM-T412. J Am Acad Dermatol 34: 244–252

Rabinovitch N, Gelfand EW, Leung DY (1999) The role of immunoglobulin therapy in allergic diseases. Allergy 54: 662–668

Richter HI, Krutmann J, Goerz G (1998) Extrakorporale Photopherese bei therapieresistentem disseminiert diskoidem Lupus erythematodes. Hautarzt 49: 487–491

Robert C, Kupper TS (1999) Inflammatory skin diseases, T cells and immune surveillance. N Engl J Med 341: 1817–1828

Roujeau JC (1999) Treatment of severe drug eruptions. J Dermatol 26: 718–722

Rzany B, Partscht K, Jung M, Kippes W, Mecking D, Baima B, Prudlo C, Pawelczyk B, Messmer EM, Schumann M, Sinkgraven R, Büchner L, Büdinger L, Pfeiffer C, Sticherling M, Hertl M, Kaiser H-W, Meurer M, Zillikens D, Messer G (2002) Risk factors for lethal outcome in patients with bullous pemphigoid. Arch Dermatol 138: 903–908

Sacher RA (2001) Intravenous immunoglobulin consensus statement. J Allergy Clin Immunol 108: 139–146

Sadayama T, Miyagawa S, Shirai T (1999) Low-dose intravenous immunoglobulin therapy for intractable dermatomyositis skin lesions. J Dermatol 26: 457–459

Saeki Y, Oshima S, Kurimoto I, Miura H, Suemura M (2000) Maintaining remission of lupus erythematosus profundus (LEP) with cyclosporin A. Lupus 9: 390–392

Sapadin AN, Fleischmajer R (2002) Treatment of scleroderma. Arch Dermatol 138: 99–105

Sauder DN (2000) Immunomodulatory and pharmacologic properties of imiquimod. J Am Acad Dermatol 43: S6–S11

Sticherling M (2001) Chronic cutaneous lupus erythematosus. In: Hertl M (ed) Autoimmune disease of the skin: pathogenesis, diagnosis, management. Springer, Wien New York, pp 169–187

Tan BB, Lear TJ, Gawkrodger DJ, English JS (1997) Azathioprine in dermatology: a survey of current practice in the UK. Br J Dermatol 136: 351–355

Thivolet J, Nicolas JF, Kanitakis J, Lyonnet S, Chouvet B (1990) Recombinant interferon alpha 2a is effective in the treatment of discoid and subacute cutaneous lupus erythematosus. Br J Dermatol 122: 405–409

Thoma-Uszynski S, Hertl M (2001) Novel therapeutic approaches in autoimmune skin disorders. In: Hertl M (ed) Autoimmune disease of the skin: pathogenesis, diagnosis, management. Springer, Wien New York, pp 337–364

Warren KJ, Nopper AJ, Crosby DL (1998) Thalidomide for recalcitrant discoid lesions in a patient with systemic lupus erythematosus. J Am Acad Dermatol 39: 293–295

Werth VP (1993) Management and treatment with systemic glucocorticoids. Adv Dermatol 8: 81–101

Wollina U, Looks A (1999) Extracorporeal photochemotherapy in cutaneous lupus erythematosus. J Eur Acad Dermatol Venereol 13: 127–130

Wozel G (1996) Dapson: Pharmakologie, Wirkmechanismus und klinischer Einsatz. Thieme, Stuttgart

Long-term effects of T cell vaccination in multiple sclerosis

**Piet Stinissen*, Guy Hermans, Niels Hellings,
Robert Medaer, and Jef Raus**

Biomedisch Onderzoeksinstituut, Limburgs Universitair Centrum, and School of Life Sciences,
Transnational University Limburg, Diepenbeek, Belgium

Introduction

Multiple sclerosis (MS) is an inflammatory disease of the central nervous system (CNS) characterised by focal areas of demyelination in the CNS (Ffrench-Constant 1994). Autoimmune processes involving myelin-reactive T cells are considered to play an essential role in the pathogenesis of MS (for a review, see Stinissen et al. 1997). In vivo activated T cells reactive to myelin basic protein (MBP) are clonally expanded in the blood of MS patients and may persist for many years in some patients (Goebels et al. 2000). The activation of MBP-reactive T cells via molecular mimicry could be a common process, as suggested by the high level of cross-reactivity of MBP-reactive T cells to various microbial ligands, even in the absence of any sequence homology (Wucherpfennig et al. 1995, Hemmer et al. 1998). Accidentally stimulated autoreactive T cells however may not automatically lead to autoimmunity. Indeed, several observations support the existence of a peripheral regulatory network that prevents activation or expansion of pathogenic T cells (Cohen et al. 1992). However, an imbalanced regulatory network may lead to suboptimal suppression of activated pathogenic T cells and give rise to autoimmunity. Administration of attenuated autoreactive T cells as a vaccine (T cell vaccination, TCV) may enhance the regulatory networks to specifically suppress the eliciting autoreactive T cells as shown in experimental autoimmune encephalomyelitis (EAE), an animal model of MS (Ben-Nun et al. 1981, Lider et al. 1988). We have performed a pilot study of TCV with MBP-reactive T cells in a small number of MS patients (Zhang et al. 1993, Medaer et al. 1995). The patients were immunised three times with autologous irradiated MBP-reactive T cell clones (see Fig. 1).

* Authors' address: Biomedisch Onderzoeksinstituut DWI, Limburgs Universitair Centrum, University Campus Building A, 3590 Diepenbeek, Belgium.
E-mail: piet.stinissen@luc.ac.be

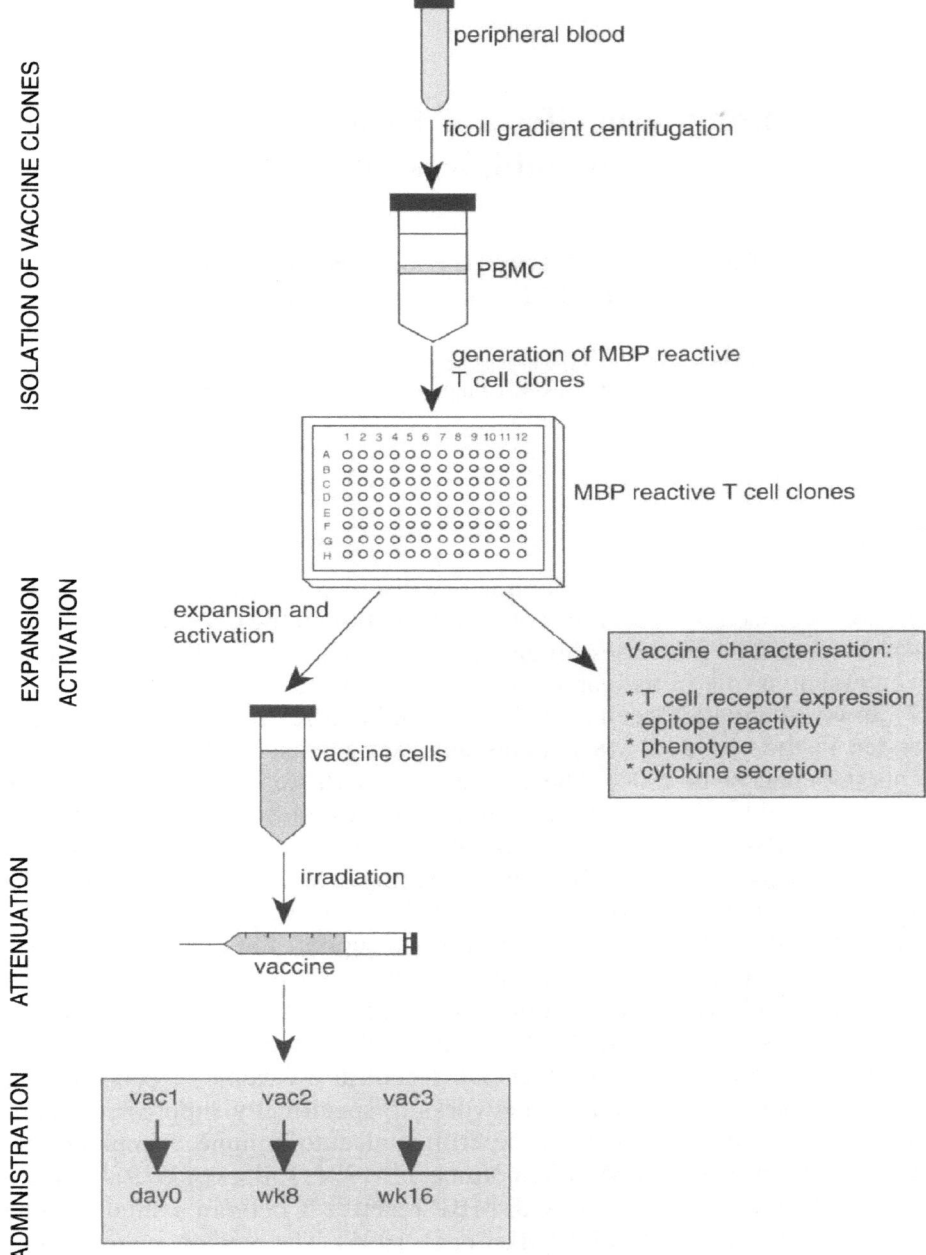

Our studies showed that CD8$^+$ anticlonotypic T cells, which specifically lyse the immunised myelin-reactive T cells in a class I-restricted fashion may play an important role in the protective mechanisms of TCV (Zhang et al. 1993, 1995).

We recently performed a follow-up study of the immunological responses to the vaccine and circulating MBP-reactive T cells in the treated patients 4–5 years after TCV (Hermans et al. 2000). These findings are summarised in the next section. In addition to its promising therapeutic application, TCV provides a unique tool to study in vivo network regulation in the normal immune system to control autoreactive T cells. Indeed, TCV may upregulate the anticlonotypic networks to control autoreactive T cells. Analysis of the antivaccine T cell responses may provide clues about the nature of the regulatory mechanisms involved. Therefore, we then discuss more recent information on the phenotypic and functional characteristics of anti-vaccine T cells isolated from the vaccinated patients (Hermans et al. 1999).

Long-term follow-up of immune responses in patients of the pilot TCV trial

There is no information about the long-term effects of TCV on the circulating myelin-reactive T cells. We have previously shown that cellular anti-vaccine responses are present in all vaccinated patients, which is associated with a specific depletion of circulating MBP-reactive T cells (Zhang et al. 1993). MBP-reactive T cells were undetectable by limiting dilution analysis in all patients (9) treated with TCV (Zhang et al. 1995). At that time it was not clear whether MBP-reactive T cells would reappear in the blood of the treated patients; and if so, whether the functional characteristics of these new clones would be different from those of the original (vaccine) clones. We therefore recently performed a follow-up evaluation of the patients who were treated with TCV. This analysis showed that in 5 of 9 MS patients MBP-reactive T cells reappeared after 1–2 years (MS7, MS8, MS9) or 3–4 years (MS4, MS3). Remarkably, the appearance of these cells coincided with clinical relapses in two of these patients (see Fig. 2) (Zhang et al. 1995). T cell receptor (TCR) analysis revealed that these clones had a clonal origin different from the T cells present before vaccination (Stinissen et al. 1997) (see Table 1).

Fig. 1. Overview of the vaccine preparation protocol used in the pilot trial. Peripheral blood mononuclear cells (PBMC) are purified from heparinized blood by Ficoll gradient centrifugation. The PBMC are plated at different cell densities and stimulated with MBP in 96-well microtiter plates. After one week, the cultures are stimulated again with MBP-pulsed antigen-presenting cells. At day 14 the cultures are screened by a classical proliferation assay, and MBP-reactive T cell lines are identified. The limiting dilution conditions allow determination of the precursor frequency of the MBP-specific T cells. MBP-reactive T cell clones are obtained by plating out the cell lines at 0.3 or 1 cell per well and stimulation with phytohemagglutinin and irradiated feeder cells. The clones obtained are characterised for their epitope reactivity and T cell receptor gene rearrangements. The selected clones are then expanded to high cell numbers (typically 40–60 million cells) by repeated stimulation with MBP-pulsed antigen-presenting cells. To prepare the cells for vaccination, the clones are activated by MBP 8 days prior to vaccination and then attenuated by irradiation (6000 rads, Cs source). The vaccine clones are injected at a dose of 10–15 million cells per clone. Three inoculations are performed with an interval of 2 months

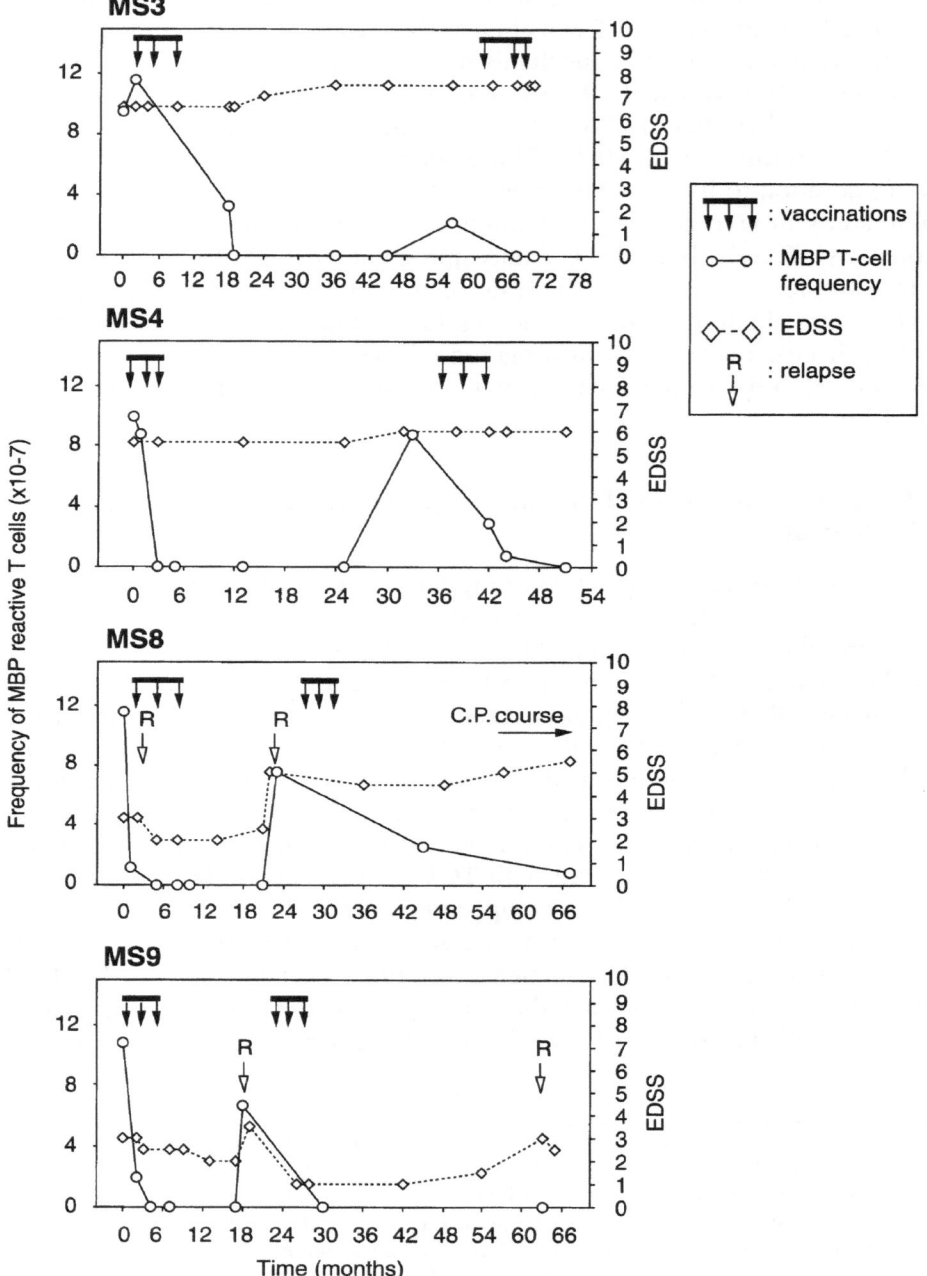

Fig. 2. Depletion of MBP-reactive T cells by additional TCV. Four MS patients with reappearing MBP-reactive T cells were revaccinated with these new MBP-reactive T cell clones. The frequency of MBP-reactive T cells was determined by limiting dilution assays at various time points before and after the second round of TCV. Each round of TCV consisted of three subsequent immunisations (2–4 month intervals) with 10 million attenuated cells of each autologous MBP-reactive clone. The patients were monitored for changes in expanded disability status score (EDSS) and relapse rate (R). One patient (MS8) entered a chronic progressive (C.P.) course at the end of the follow-up period

Table 1. Cytokine pattern, TCR expression, and epitope specificity of MBP-reactive T cells isolated before and after T cell vaccination

Patient	Clone	Isolation	TCR expression[a]			Cytokine production (pg/ml)[b]						Epitope reactivity
			SI[c]	AV–AJ	BV–BJ	IFN-γ	IL-4	IL-2	TNF-α	IL-10	TGF-β	
MS9	D7	Pre-TCV	46.8	13.1–57	5–2.4	2599	60	1457	84	0	0	84–102
	1B7	Post-TCV	209.1	22–37	13.1–1.2	240	0	272	81	10	0	61–82
	2C3	Post-TCV	16.2	22–37	13.1–1.2	270	0	169	52	13	0	61–82
	2F10	Post-TCV	63.4	NT[d]	6.6–1.2	0	0	270	39	6	0	84–102
	2C5	Post-TCV	44.2	14.1–34	13.1–1.1	300	0	203	66	8	0	124–142
MS3[e]	5	Pre-TCV	89.3	10	5	7540	0	1404	246	185	44	45–89
	E4	Pre-TCV	2.3	12	2	2253	0	339	210	118	46	143–168
	2E6	Post-TCV	2.7	13.1–22	4.1–1.2	5519	6	4598	183	36	81	84–102
MS4	2F7	Pre-TCV	216.7	10.1–42	7.1–2.7	1420	0	1456	366	22	9	84–102
	1E3	Pre-TCV	149.2	15.1–38	7.2–2.1	1180	33	2176	332	27	0	NI[f]
	3B1	Pre-TCV	41.0	15.1–38	7.2–2.1	1200	134	1738	332	6	0	NI
	2C8	Post-TCV	20.0	9.1–x	1.1–2.7	1090	0	760	254	4	8	NI
	2E2	Post-TCV	28.6	1.4–57	13.1–2.3	1280	0	420	293	49	0	NI
	1G5	Post-TCV	42.0	1.4–16	13.1–1.2	0	0	169	95	5	0	NI
	2D2	Post-TCV	7.9	6.1–7	17.1–2.7	340	0	59	99	0	0	61–82
	2D6	Post-TCV	2.4	1.4–57	13.1–2.3	2440	6	1446	675	0	40	NI

[a] T cell receptor variable (V) and joining (J) gene usage of the α-chain (A) and β-chain (B)

[b] Net cytokine concentration in conditioned supernatant

[c] Stimulation index

[d] Not tested

[e] For the clones MS3-5 and MS3-E4 only TCR AV and BV gene usage are listed (CDR3 sequence analysis was not done)

[f] Not identified; the clones responded to stimulation with MBP but not to any of the synthetic peptides tested

MBP-reactive T cell clones isolated before and after TCV possess similar functional properties

We studied whether the new MBP-reactive T cells identified after TCV express the same functional properties as those isolated before treatment. This is an important question because it relates to the potential pathogenicity of these cells in the disease process. The cytokine profile, cytotoxic potential, and epitope reactivity of the MBP-reactive T cell clones isolated after vaccination were studied and compared with the properties of the original isolates. The MBP-reactive T cells isolated before and after TCV produced mixed cytokine patterns resembling a Th0-like pattern with high levels of gamma interferon (IFN-γ), interleukin-2 (IL-2), and tumor necrosis factor alpha (TNFα). IL-4, IL-10, and transforming growth factor (TGF-β) were produced by a small number of clones and in low quantities (Table 1). In patient MS9, a slightly different cytokine production pattern was observed for the clones isolated after TCV as compared to the clone used for vaccination (D7). Production of IL-4 was detected in the vaccine clone but not in the post-TCV clones. The levels of IFN-γ production by the post-TCV clones were only about one tenth of the IFN-γ production of the vaccine clone. In contrast, low levels of IL-10 were produced by the post-TCV clones but not by the clone used in the vaccine. Analysis of the epitope reactivity of these clones showed a diverse pattern of epitope specificity for the clones isolated after TCV (Table 1). One of the post-TCV clones (2F10) had the same peptide reactivity (84–102) as the vaccine clone. All clones showed cytotoxic reactivity against MBP-pulsed autologous target cells. The post-TCV clones had a clonal origin different from the vaccine clone as illustrated by a different TCR AV-AJ and BV-BJ usage (Table 1).

In patient MS3, the two clones isolated before and the single clone isolated after TCV had a similar cytokine profile, expressing high levels of IFN-γ, IL-2, TNF-α. These clones produced little or no IL-4, but substantial amounts of IL-10 and TGF-β. The clone isolated after TCV recognised the immunodominant 84–102 epitope, which was not recognised by the two vaccine clones, and had a TCR AV and BV usage different from the vaccine clones. The clones of patient MS4 produced a rather heterogeneous pattern of cytokines. The three clones isolated before TCV produced high levels of IFN-γ, IL-2, and TNF-α, but two clones also produced IL-4 and IL-10. The clones isolated after vaccination generally had a similar cytokine production pattern, although one clone did not produce IFN-γ. Most of these post-TCV clones did not produce IL-4, while some produced IL-10 or TGF-β. One of the post-TCV clones and one of the vaccine clones were tested for cytotoxicity but did not lyse the MBP-pulsed target cells. Interestingly, most of the clones of this patient did not recognise any of the overlapping peptides tested, although they showed high proliferative responses to MBP (Table 1). The post-TCV clones had a clonal origin different from the clones isolated before TCV as shown by different TCR V gene usage (Table 1).

The data suggest that the MBP clones isolated before and after TCV possess similar functional reactivities. Although the relevance of the cytotoxic potential of MBP-reactive T cells in the pathogenesis of MS is not clear, some of the clones isolated before or after TCV show cytotoxic reactivity against MBP-pulsed targets. These clones also express a similar Th0-like cytokine production pattern. Clearly the clones did not shift towards a Th2 or Th3 phenotype after TCV as observed in other treatments (Hafler et al. 1997, Waisman et al. 1996). It is possible that the in vitro culturing steps may have influenced the cytokine pattern of the clones. This seems however unlikely since we and others have shown that the cytokine production profile of MBP-reactive T cell clones remains stable during T cell culture and is comparable with the profile of short-term MBP-reactive T cell lines (Hermans et al. 1997, Hemmer et al. 1996). On the basis of studies of the encephalitogenic T cells in EAE, it has been suggested that myelin-reactive T cells which produce proinflammatory cytokines and recognise the immunodominant regions of MBP may be pathogenic in MS (for a review, see Stinissen et al. 1998a). If this holds true, our data indicate that some of the MBP-reactive T cell clones isolated after TCV may play a role in the perpetuation of the disease process. This is in line with our previous observations showing a correlation between the reappearance of MBP-reactive T cells and worsening of the disease process in some patients (Zhang et al. 1995).

Reappearing MBP-reactive T cell clones can be depleted by additional sequence of vaccinations

Because our results suggest that the reappearing clones may potentially have pathogenic properties, it was decided to revaccinate four patients with a vaccine consisting of these new clones. Three vaccinations were performed by essentially the same protocol as for the initial TCV treatment (Fig. 1), and MBP-reactive T cell frequencies were determined by limiting dilution analysis. As shown in Fig. 2, revaccination of patients MS3, MS4, MS8, and MS9 was followed by a gradual decrease in the frequency of MBP-reactive T cells. In 3 of 4 patients, no MBP-reactive T cells were isolated after this second round of TCV. Overall the frequency decreased less rapidly than was observed after the first TCV treatment. As for the initial TCV treatment, no adverse effects were observed in these patients after revaccination. The analysis of the expanded disability status score (EDSS) and relapses before and after this second round of TCV suggests that the vaccinations did not induce clinical worsening in these patients (Fig. 1). The revaccinated patients are currently monitored to examine whether new anti-MBP reactivity will appear in these patients. These results demonstrate that it is feasible to deplete the reappearing clones successfully in a second round of TCV.

Long-term follow-up: concluding remarks

Circulating MBP-reactive T cells were not detected in the majority of TCV-treated patients 1 to 2 years after TCV. It remains unknown whether the clones are depleted from the circulation or became anergised after TCV and can therefore no longer be isolated by stimulation with MBP. MBP T cells reappeared in 5 patients after an additional period of 1 to 3 years. The reappearing clones have similar functional characteristics but belong to a different clonal origin as those isolated before TCV. It is possible that the reappearing clones were present cryptically before TCV, when the MBP-specific repertoire was dominated by other clones, but became activated during a new priming event. This event may be related to epitope-spreading mechanisms as observed in EAE (Lehmann et al. 1993). Likewise, these clones may have been activated by cross-reactive epitopes of viral or bacterial antigens with a homology with MBP (Wucherpfennig et al. 1995). Interestingly, despite the reappearance of new clones in some patients, the original clones remained undetected in all patients for at least 5 years after TCV. This suggests that the clonotype-specific immune responses raised against the original vaccine clones after the first TCV were sufficient to induce long-term depletion.

Our data further demonstrate that TCV induces long-term immune responses in a clonotype specific manner. While this response may be sufficient to deplete anti-MBP T cell reactivity in a subgroup of patients, the dynamic properties of the autoreactive T cell repertoire may lead to in vivo activation of cryptic anti-MBP clones in other patients. These clones can however be depleted in subsequent rounds of TCV. These data suggest that it may not be sufficient to knock out the autoreactive T cell clones at a given time point to prevent autoreactive T cell responses at later stages in the disease process. Thus, our findings are of importance not only for the design of further TCV trials but also for other T-cell-targeted immunotherapies as treatments for MS and other T-cell-mediated autoimmune diseases.

Analysis of cellular and humoral responses to the vaccine cells in T-cell-vaccinated patients

We have previously shown that CD8 anticlonotypic T cells specific for the vaccine cells can be identified after TCV (Zhang et al. 1993). However, it is possible that other T lymphocytes are involved in the suppression or down-regulation of auto-reactive T cells after TCV. For instance, $\gamma\delta$ T cells respond to the vaccine cells and may play a role in the regulation of autoreactive T cells by T cell-to-T cell inter-actions or by the secretion of soluble factors (Stinissen et al. 1998b). To character-ise the T cell and antibody responses that are induced by TCV, these studies were extended in a group of 49 MS patients who were recently treated with TVC. This study was performed to determine the safety, immune responses, and clinical effects in a larger group of patients (Stinissen et al. 1998c). The phenotype, cytokine secre-tion profile, and functional properties of the T cells that were reactive to the vaccine cells were evaluated. To this end, peripheral blood lymphocytes were stimulated with irradiated T cell clones and both cells and supernatant were harvested for further evaluation (Fig. 3).

Characteristics of antivaccine cells: phenotype and functional properties

Phenotype

To provide additional information on cell subsets which respond to the vaccine clones, the phenotypic characteristics of the cultures, obtained by stimulation of peripheral blood monocytes (PBMC) with the irradiated vaccine cells, were evalu-ated. Cultures were harvested at day 7 and analysed with a fluorescence-activated cell sorter. Figure 4 shows the results of experiments where PBMC of three vacci-nated patients were analysed 4 weeks after the third vaccination. Proliferative responses induced by the immunising clones but also T cell blasts stimulated by phytohemagglutinin (PHA) were observed in all patients with stimulation index (SI) values ranging from 2.1 to 21.5. The vaccine cells induced expansions of a heterogeneous mixture of cell subsets. In patients MED and THD the vaccine clones primarily stimulated CD8$^+$ T cells, but also CD4$^+$ cells and in addition double-negative cells were observed after stimulation. The phenotype of the responding cells was slightly different when different vaccine clones were used as stimulus. In patient DM about one third of the cells were CD4$^+$, one third was CD8$^+$, while the remaining fraction was CD4$^-$CD8$^-$. The majority of cells were TCR$\alpha\beta^+$, although in some cases up to 10% of the responding cells were TCR$\gamma\delta^+$, which is in line with our previous observations (Stinissen et al. 1998b). All tested clones stimulated NK cells (CD3$^-$CD16/56$^+$). No correlation was found between the level of the proliferative response and the resulting phenotypic profile. In summary, the in vitro T cell response to the vaccine was dominated by TCR$\alpha\beta^+$

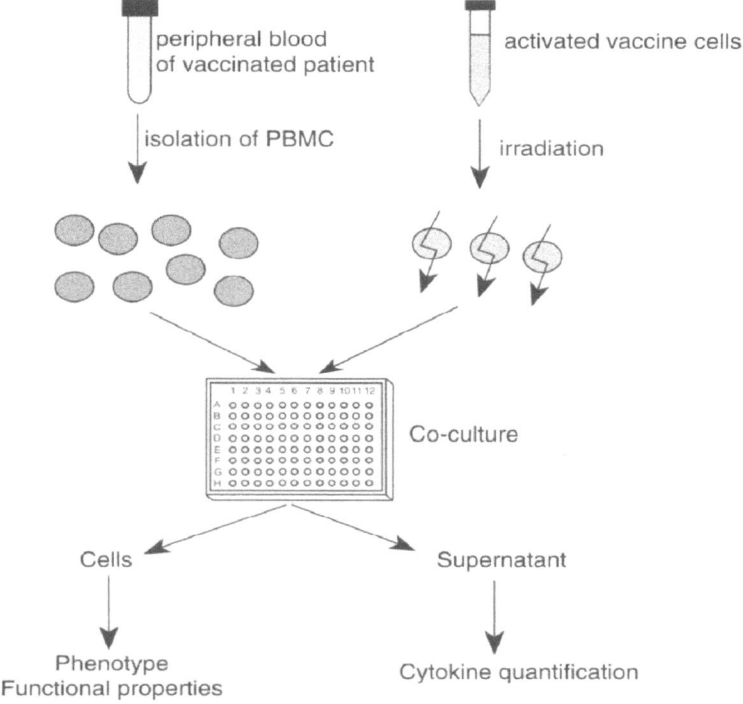

Fig. 3. In vitro antivaccine assays. PBMC of vaccinated patients were collected at various time intervals before and after vaccinations and stimulated with irradiated activated T cell clones (vaccine cells). Cells were harvested at day 4 and the incorporated radioactivity was determined to evaluate the vaccine-induced in vitro proliferation of PBMC. The supernatant of these cultures was used for cytokine quantification by an enzyme-linked immunosorbent assay. Parallel cultures were harvested at day 7 to determine the phenotype of the responding lymphocytes

of mainly CD8 and CD4 phenotype, although also TCRγδ$^+$ and NK cells are present in the vaccine-stimulated cultures.

Specific cytotoxicity and inhibition

Cell subsets among the heterogeneous short-term antivaccine lines were studied for their ability to induce either cytolysis or direct inhibition of the proliferation of the vaccine clones. To determine the relative contribution of anti-clonotypic T cells among the heterogeneous T cell lines derived by stimulating PBMC with the vaccine cells, the lines were cloned by limiting dilution with PHA and the resulting clones were tested for their ability to specifically inhibit or lyse the original vaccine clone used for primary stimulation (Table 2). The phenotype of the original lines was: line 2D5 (DM-PBMC stimulated with clone DM-2D5): 31% CD4$^+$, 37% CD8$^+$, 26% CD4$^-$CD8$^-$; line 2D6 (DM-PBMC stimulated with clone DM-2D6): 28% CD4$^+$, 37% CD8$^+$, 28% CD4$^-$CD8$^-$. Although the initial lines had a mixed phenotype of CD4$^+$ and CD8$^+$ but also CD4$^-$CD8$^-$, the majority of the resulting

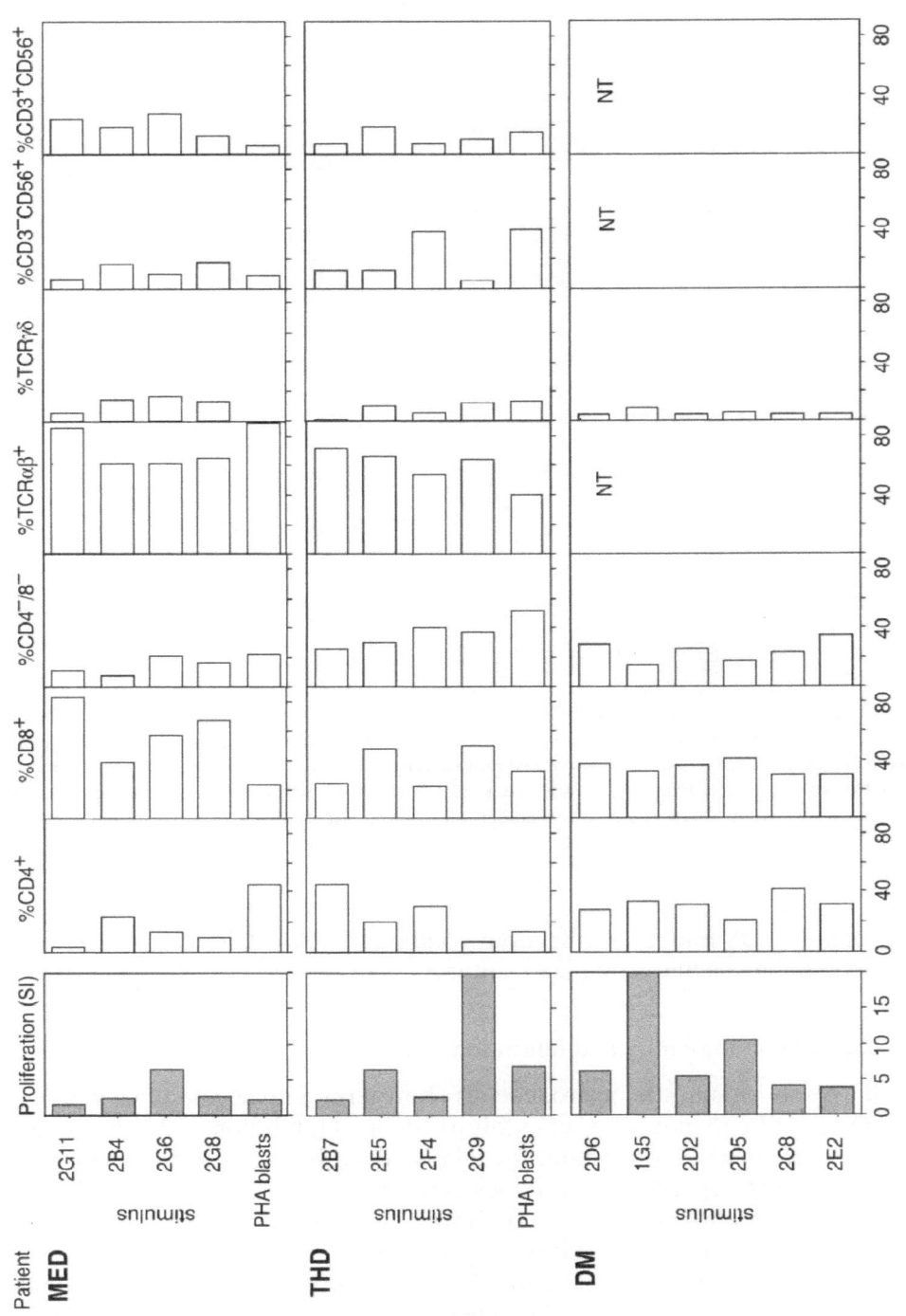

Table 2. Characteristics of T cell clones obtained by cloning the T cell lines responding to stimulation with the vaccine clones[a]

Original stimulus of PBMC	Nr. of resulting clones of phenotype:			Nr. of clones inducing:[b]			
	CD4+	CD8+	CD4−CD8−	cytolysis		inhibition	
				CD4	CD8	CD4	CD8
DM-2D5	25/38	13/38	0/38	0/8	1/11a	0/8	1/11a
DM-2D6	21/38	13/38	0/38	0/10	2/8b	0/10	2/8b

[a] PBMC of patient DM (isolated 4 weeks after the third vaccination) were stimulated with one of the T cell clones used for vaccination (DM2-D5 and DM-2D6) and phenotypically analysed on day 7. The phenotype of the resulting lines was: DM-PBMC + DM-2D5: 31% CD4+, 37% CD8+, and 26% CD4−CD8−; DM-PBMC + DM-2D6: 28% CD4+, 37% CD8+, and 26% CD4−CD8−. On the same day, the lines were cloned by stimulation with PHA and irradiated feeder cells at single-cell densities, and resulting clones were expanded on IL-2. The clones were then tested for CD4 and CD8 expression with a fluorescence-activated cell sorter and a randomly selected fraction of the clones was tested for specific cytotoxic recognition of the original stimulator clone in a standard chromium-release assay (scored positive if more than 20% specific release was observed). The clones were also tested for their ability to inhibit the antigen-specific proliferation of the original stimulator clone (scored positive if more than 50% inhibition was observed). For the latter experiment 2×10^4 vaccine clone T cells were stimulated with 5×10^5 MBP-pulsed antigen-presenting cells, and 4×10^4 irradiated antivaccine clone cells were added
[b] Identical letters following values indicate that the same clones were cytolytic and inhibitory

clones were CD4+ and a smaller number of clones were CD8+. However, no CD4−CD8− clones were obtained, suggesting that the cloning procedure was biased towards the growth of these two subsets. Interestingly, none of the CD4+ clones did recognise the original vaccine clone in a cytolytic or inhibition assay. Among the CD8+ clones tested, some clones (2 of 8 for 2D6, and 1 of 11 for 2D5) expressed a typical anti-clonotypic recognition profile (Fig. 5). In summary, although different lymphocyte cell subsets responded to stimulation with the vaccine clones, after cloning, only a small number of CD8+ clones was able to specifically recognise the original stimulating clone.

Cytokine secretion

The cytokine profile of the T cells responding to in vitro stimulation with the vaccine cells may provide information on the type of immune response that is

Fig. 4. Phenotypic profile of short-term cell lines derived by stimulation with vaccine clones. PBMC of vaccinated patients were obtained 4 weeks after vaccination 3 and stimulated with irradiated vaccine clones or with irradiated autologous PHA-stimulated T cell blasts. Cells were harvested at day 4, and the incorporated radioactivity (counts per minute) was determined. The stimulation index (SI) was calculated by division of the counts per minute of the combination of PBMC plus vaccine clone through the sum of the counts per minute of the vaccine clone alone and of the PBMC alone. At day 7 the cells were stained with fluorescently labelled antibody pairs and analysed by flow cytometry. Results are presented as percent staining with the respective antibody

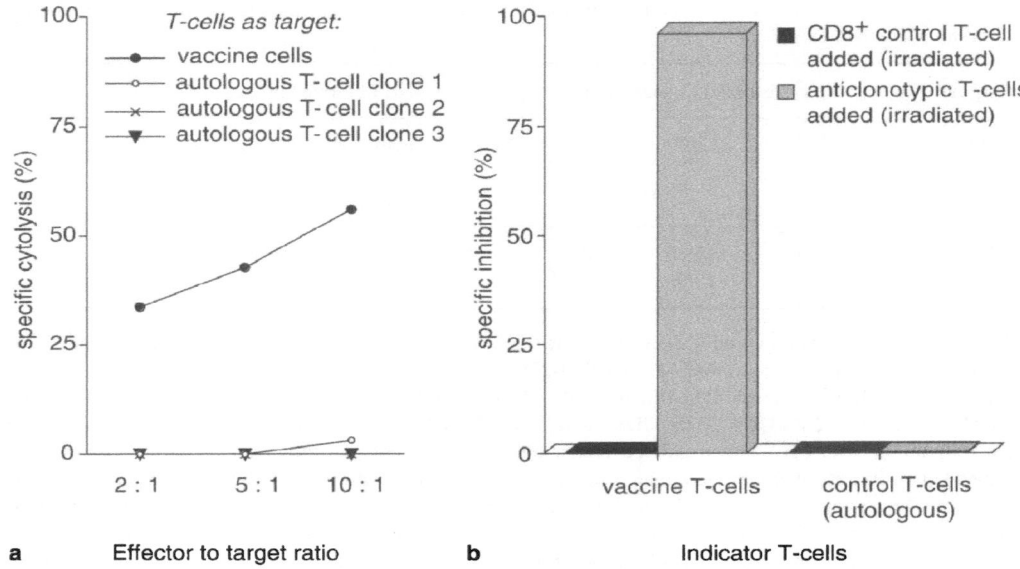

Fig. 5. Cytotoxic (**a**) and inhibitory (**b**) properties of CD8⁺ anticlonotypic T cell clones isolated from vaccinated MS patients. CD8 anticlonotypic T cell clones were isolated from PBMC of vaccinated patients by repeated stimulation with irradiated vaccine cells. The anticlonotypic T cells specifically lyse the vaccine clones but no other autologous T cell clones with different TCRs (**a**). The anticlonotypic T cells are also able to specifically suppress the MBP-induced proliferation of vaccine clones (**b**)

predominantly generated by TCV: T1, T2, or a mixed T0-like response. We collected supernatant from the PBMC cultures stimulated with the irradiated vaccine clones after 72 h of stimulation and analysed the levels of IFN-γ, IL-4, IL-2, TNF-α, and IL-10 by an enzyme-linked immunosorbent assay. As a control we also studied the cytokine production of unstimulated PBMC and of irradiated vaccine cells incubated separately. Nonstimulated PBMC did not produce any IL-4, but in some cases low levels of IFN-γ were detected (<50 pg/ml). Irradiated vaccine clones frequently produced low levels (<20 pg/ml) of IFN-γ, TNF-α, IL-10, and IL-2. The cytokine production of these control cultures was subtracted from the values for the stimulated cultures (PBMC plus vaccine cells) to yield the net production of cytokines. Figure 6 shows the results obtained from 4 vaccinated MS patients. IFN-γ and TNF-α production was observed in most cultures. After the third vaccination the IFN-γ production was increased in most patients as compared to the production before vaccination. IL-2 production was present in a limited number of assays only. Low levels of IL-10 were observed frequently after the first and second vaccination, but they decreased after the third vaccination. IL-4 production was observed in one patient (MIV) only but was clearly clone dependent. Only stimulation with clone MIV-2G4 induced IL-4 production, while other vaccine clones of the same patient (2F10, 2E8, 2B7) did not. The levels of cytokines produced did not correlate with the levels of the proliferative responses. For instance, 4 weeks after the second vaccination clone 2F10 of patient MIV induced a strong proliferation with an SI of 43 but a relatively low IFN-γ production

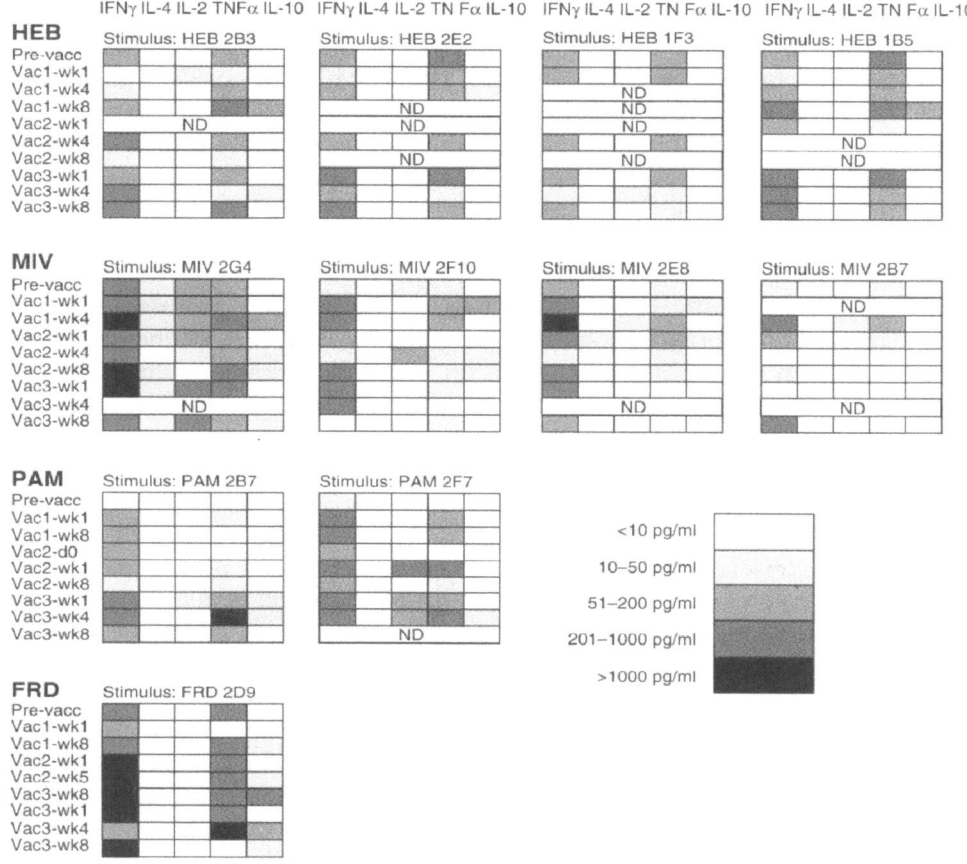

Fig. 6. Cytokine production profile of short-term cell lines derived by stimulation with vaccine clones. PBMC of vaccinated patients were collected at various time points before and after vaccinations and stimulated with irradiated vaccine clones. As a control, irradiated stimulator cells alone and PBMC alone were plated in culture medium. Cell supernatants were harvested at day 4 and cytokine production was measured by an enzyme-linked immunosorbent assay. The net cytokine release was calculated by subtraction of the background cytokine release (release from PBMC alone and irradiated stimulator cells alone) from the release of the stimulated cultures (PBMC plus stimulus)

(39 pg/ml), while the same clone induced less proliferation 1 week after vaccination 3 (SI = 4) but high IFN-γ production (676 pg/ml).

In summary, the antivaccine T cells predominantly produced proinflammatory cytokines IFN-γ and TNF-α, although low levels of IL-10 were also detected. One vaccine clone induced IL-4 only, suggesting that the production of this cytokine relates to an unknown characteristic expressed by this autoreactive T cell clone. We also performed some experiments to test which cell types were responsible for the cytokine production. CD8+ cells, CD4+ cells, or γδ T cells were depleted from the PBMC by antibody-coated magnetic beads. The depleted cell mixtures were stimulated in vitro with irradiated vaccine cells. At day 4 of incubation, cell proliferation was measured and culture supernatants were harvested for cytokine analysis. Depletion of CD4 cells most often reduced the proliferation upon stimulation with vaccine clones. Depletion of $CD8^+$ T cells did not significantly alter the proliferation, while $\gamma\delta$ T cell depletion led to an increased proliferative activity in some cases. Furthermore, cytokine production was mainly affected by depletion of the $CD4^+$ subset, while depletion of $CD8^+$ and $\gamma\delta$ T cells had little or no effect on the overall cytokine production. Interestingly, the IL-4 production, which was observed only in patient MIV after stimulation with clone MIV-2G4, was almost completely abolished after depletion of the CD4 subset. The same observation was made for the IL-10 production. Although $\gamma\delta$ T cell depletion most often increased proliferation as compared to nondepleted PBMC, the depletion of these cells did not have a major effect on cytokine production. In conclusion, $CD4^+$ T cells predominantly contributed to the cytokine production induced by stimulation with the vaccine clones.

Antibody responses to the vaccine clones after vaccination

In view of the observations that antilymphocyte antibodies play a major role in the protective effects of T cell vaccination in EAE (Herkel et al. 1997), an evaluation was made of the humoral responses to vaccine cells in patients treated with TCV. The presence of antibodies which could either bind to living vaccine cells (by flow cytometry) or bind to protein extracts made from vaccine clones (by Western blotting) was evaluated in serum of the vaccinated patients. Furthermore, the effects of serum on antigen-specific proliferation of the vaccine clones were studied.

When vaccine clones and/or PHA-stimulated T cells were incubated with the serum samples and antibody binding was evaluated by flow cytometry, only low staining percentages were observed (Table 3). In one patient an increased staining was observed after vaccination 2 (3.4%) which further increased to 9.7% one week after vaccination 3 but returned to baseline values 3 weeks later. In this patient the staining was rather specific for the immunising clone as less staining was observed with PHA-stimulated T cell blasts. Overall, serum staining was very low as compared to 74–95% staining of vaccine clones in vaccinated Lewis rats (Herkel et al. 1997). Immunoblotting analysis (in collaboration with Dr. A. Lohse, Mainz) of sera from vaccinated patients showed reactivity to several proteins, but there was no difference in the staining pattern obtained before and after vaccination. Finally, serum of the vaccinated patients was tested for the presence of antibodies or other components that specifically inhibit the proliferation of the vaccine clones as observed in Lewis rats. On the basis of the flow-cytometric data, serum from patient INE (no staining) and INC (moderate staining after vaccination 3) were selected for these experiments. As demonstrated in Fig. 7, serum samples of patient INE did not affect the proliferation of the vaccine clones INE-2C8 and INE-1F8. INC serum showed a slight inhibition (19%) after the first and second vaccinations but a much higher inhibition (78%) 1 week after vaccination 3, corresponding to the increased staining as observed by flow cytometry. Again, 4 weeks after vaccination 3 the inhibition disappeared. Although this inhibition may have been caused by

Table 3. Positive staining (percentage) of vaccine clones by serum antibodies from the vaccinated patients[a]

Patient	Cells stained	% staining of T cells with serum					
		control (FCS)	before vac	1 wk after vac1	1 wk after vac2	1 wk after vac3	4 wks after vac3
INC	INC-2F8	0.4	1.1	0.5	3.4	9.7	1.2
	PHA blasts	0.1	0.1	0	1.1	2.1	3.4
CAD	CAD-2C4	0.2	0	0	0.1	2.9	NT
	CAD-2G4	0	0	0	0.1	3.4	NT
	PHA blasts	0	0	0	0	4.8	NT
HEB	HEB-2B3	0.6	0.4	0.3	0.5	1.0	0.2
	HEB-1F3	0	0.9	0.7	0.1	0.8	0.1
	PHA blasts	0.2	0	0.2	0	0	0.1
FRD	FRD-2D9	0.2	1.9	1.0	0	0.6	0
	PHA blasts	0	1.3	2.2	0.2	0.9	0.6
INE	INE-1E11	0	0.9	0.4	0.6	0	0.6
	INE-1F8	3.3	0.6	0.2	0.4	1.5	3.3
	INE-2C8	0	1.0	3.6	0	0.2	0.2

[a] Cells were incubated with 25% (v/v) of serum from vaccinated patients or fetal calf serum (FCS) as a control for 1 h and subsequently stained with fluorescein isothiocyanate-labelled goat anti-human immunoglobulin G/A/M secondary antibody. Cells stained with the secondary antibody alone were used as control to define background staining

other components such as cytokines, the correlation with the flow-cytometric data suggests that antibodies may have participated in this inhibition. In conclusion, no major antibody responses towards the vaccine clones were observed in the vaccinated patients. In one patient, inhibiting antibodies to the vaccine cells were observed 1 week after the third vaccination, but these antibodies disappeared 3 weeks later.

Antivaccine responses in T-cell-vaccinated patients: concluding remarks

Little is known about the mechanism of TCV in MS. We have previously described both anti-clonotypic and anti-ergotypic T cell responses to the vaccine clones in vaccinated patients. Anti-clonotypic T cells were mainly CD8[+] T cells which expressed cytotoxic and inhibitory reactivity towards the vaccine clones in a major histocompatibility complex (MHC) class I-restricted manner (Zhang et al. 1993, 1995). Here additional information on the cellular and antibody responses to the vaccine clones provides further insight into the mechanisms of TCV. Significant antivaccine responses were observed in PBMC of the vaccinated patients. In the majority of patients a maximal proliferative response was observed after the second vaccination. SI values higher than 10 were observed, suggesting a strong immune response to the vaccine. Vigorous secondary immune responses towards vaccines are generally ascribed to expanded vaccine-responsive memory cell

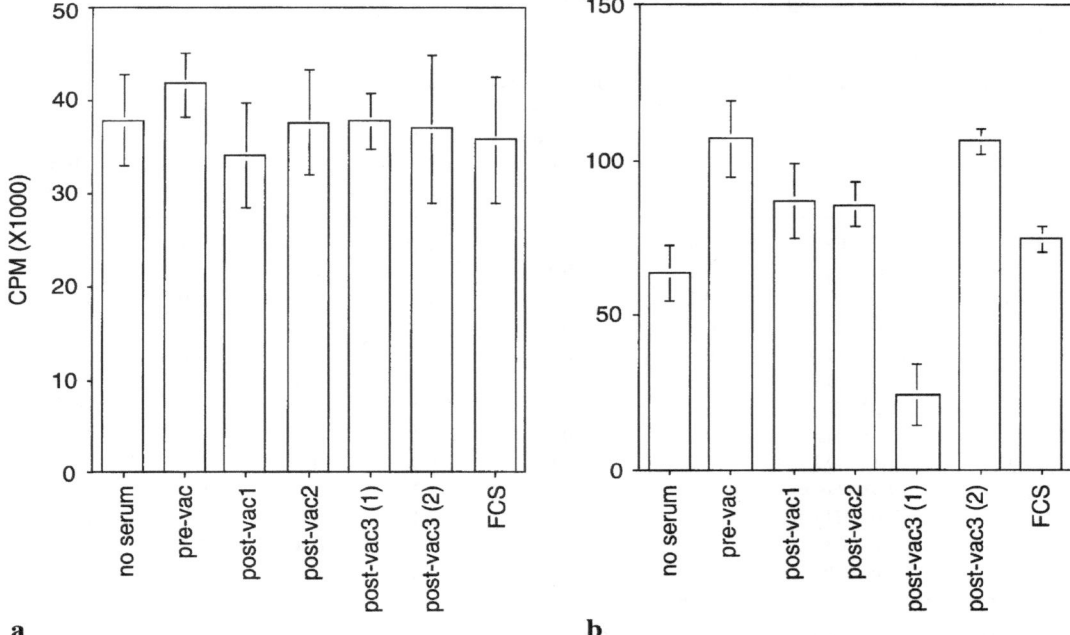

Fig. 7a, b. Proliferation of vaccine T cell clones INE-2C8 (**a**) and INC-2F8 (**b**) stimulated with MBP-pulsed irradiated PBMC in the presence or absence of serum from vaccinated patients. Vaccine T cell clones were stimulated with irradiated autologous PBMC only or MBP-pulsed irradiated PBMC as antigen-presenting cells in the presence of 10% autologous serum obtained before vaccination (*pre-vac*), 1 week after vaccination 1, 2, or 3 (*post-vac1, post-vac2, post-vac3(1)*), or 4 weeks after vaccination 3 (*post-vac3(2)*), or 10% fetal calf serum (*FCS*). Three wells were plated for each serum sample. As a control, cultures were set up with-out serum. ³H-thymidine was added after three days of incubation and cells were harvested 16 h later. The incorporated radioactivity (counts per minute, ×1000) is presented as mean with standard deviation. The background incorporation of the T cell clones was 542 and 5,726 cpm for the clones INE-2C8 and INC-2F8 respectively

populations. If this holds true for TCV, an important part of the enhanced immune response may relate to memory antigen-specific lymphocytes. These long-lived memory cells may account for the long half-life of the antivaccine responses. The phenotypic characteristics of the cultures obtained by stimulation with the vaccine cells demonstrated that $CD4^+$ T cells, $CD8^+$ T cells but also $CD4^-CD8^-$ cells respond to the vaccine. Although the majority of these cells were $TCR\alpha\beta^+$, short-term lines also consisted of $TCR\gamma\delta^+$ T cells and NK cells. The observation of the mixed phenotypic profile of these antivaccine lines raises two important questions: which is the antigen or stimulating factor responsible for the proliferation of these various subsets, and which of these subsets plays a role in the mechanisms of TCV?

It can be speculated that the TCR of the vaccine clones is an important target for some of the antivaccine cells. We have previously shown that $CD8^+$ anti-clonotypic T cells can be directly stimulated by the vaccine clones in a class I-restricted manner, most likely by recognition of a TCR-related sequence (Zhang et al. 1993). In addition, Vandenbark et al. (1996) have demonstrated that CD4$^+$ T cells can be stimulated by TCR peptides presented in the context of MHC class II molecules. The CD4$^+$ antivaccine lines therefore may be stimulated by TCR antigens presented by the vaccine T cells through nonclassical pathways, or through extracellular re-uptake of endogenously synthesised epitopes by T cells or other antigen-presenting cells such as the Langerhans cells in the skin (Kozovska et al. 1996). Some of the responding cells may represent anti-ergotypic cells and could be stimulated by an unknown marker commonly expressed on the surface of activated T cells (Lohse et al. 1989, 1993). We have previously shown that γδ T cells may be part of this anti-ergotypic response (Stinissen et al. 1998b). Cytokine receptors were identified as candidate targets of anti-ergotypic T cell-to-T cell interactions (Mor et al. 1996). The NK cells observed in the antivaccine cultures may play an important role in the induction of the cytotoxic-T-lymphocyte response as suggested by Kos and Engleman (1996). Finally, it is possible that some of the cells responding to stimulation with the vaccine cells are merely stimulated through bystander activation via the local release of proinflammatory cytokines.

Our data show that only among the TCRαβ$^+$ CD8$^+$ clones specific cytolytic and inhibitory reactivities towards the vaccine were observed. Although a large proportion of CD4$^+$ and CD8$^+$ clones did not display cytolytic or inhibitory anti-clonotypic reactivity towards the vaccine cells, the possibility that our cloning procedure is biased towards the isolation of clones with good growth characteristics cannot be ruled out. It is possible that regulatory cells with poor growth potential were missed. The production of anti-inflammatory cytokines could be another mechanism by which antivaccine cells may down-regulate autoreactive T cells. Therefore the cytokine production induced by stimulation with the vaccine clones in the short-term cultures was analysed. Despite the low level of IL-10 that was produced in some patients, stimulation with the vaccine clones predominantly induced production of Th1-type cytokines. Bystander-mediated suppression through the induction of anti-inflammatory cytokines is probably not a predominant mechanism of TCV. Depletion of the CD4$^+$ T cells leads to a substantial reduction of both proliferative response and cytokine production of the antivaccine lines, suggesting that CD4$^+$ T cells play a predominant role in the in vitro responses to the vaccine cells. Interestingly, the antivaccine CD4$^+$ T cells seen in our primary cultures seem to be different from those obtained after treatment with TCR peptides (Vandenbark et al. 1996). The anti-TCR peptide T cells described by Vandenbark and co-workers produced high levels of IL-10 and may induce bystander suppression as demonstrated in in vitro experiments (Vandenbark et al. 1996). The Th1-type antivaccine T cells may however correlate with the CD4 TCR-peptide-specific regulatory T cells described by Kumar and Sercarz (1998). These authors showed that priming of type 1 TCR-peptide-reactive regulatory T cells leads to the deviation of MBP-specific T cells in a type 2 direction and protection from EAE in B10.PL mice, whereas induction of type 2 regulatory cells results in exacerbation of EAE.

A low level of antibody reactivity against the vaccine was found in one patient only, which means that the humoral responses are clearly less important in TCV as compared to the antivaccine antibody responses in EAE. By flow-cytometry we never observed more than 10% of staining of the vaccine cells with serum from vaccinated patients, while in EAE more than 90% of the vaccine cells were stained with postvaccination serum (Herkel et al. 1997). The high level of vaccine staining in EAE corresponded to an increased reactivity in immunoblotting experiments, which again was not observed in the human postvaccination sera. Further studies need to resolve whether different routes of administration cause the discrepancies between the human and animal experiments, and whether the use of adjuvants would increase the antibody responses against the vaccine in the patients. However, the successful depletion of autoreactive T cells even in the absence of an efficient antibody response suggests that humoral responses to TCV are not necessary to induce effects in humans.

In summary, our data suggest that $TCR\alpha\beta^+$ $CD8^+$ T cells display direct anti-idiotypic effects towards the vaccine clones, while $CD4^+$ T cells are the predominant cytokine producers upon stimulation with the vaccine cells. Several uncommon lymphocyte populations including $\gamma\delta$ T cells and NK cells are also expanded upon stimulation with T cell vaccines, suggesting that these cells may play a role in immunoregulatory T cell-to-T cell interactions. Further studies are necessary to resolve which of these lymphocyte populations plays the most important role in the TCV mechanism. The present study provides further information on the immune response against attenuated autoreactive T cells used as a vaccine.

Future directions

Our pilot studies with TCV in MS have shown that this approach is feasible and safe in human patients. The vaccine clones appear to be immunogenic and induce an upregulation of the anti-clonotypic network. The ongoing clinical trials in our laboratory and other centres will further teach us how these regulatory networks operate to control autoreactive T cells in humans. Double-blinded, placebo-controlled clinical studies are necessary to demonstrate the clinical efficacy of TCV in MS. However, the application of T cell vaccination on a large scale is limited. Some of these limitations are summarised below.

Dose, attenuation protocol, number of vaccinations. The dose used in our pilot study (10–15 million cells of each clone) induced an antivaccine response in all patients. It remains to be studied whether smaller doses would induce the same effects of the vaccine cells as the ones observed. In addition, we do not know whether other attenuation protocols would give rise to the same effects. We have used 3 consecutive injections in each vaccination. We know that at least in some patients this is not sufficient to deplete all circulating MBP-reactive T cells. It is not clear whether as many clones as possible should be included in the vaccine or whether the most active ones at a particular time should be included. The latter procedure most likely would result in repeated vaccinations.

Repeated vaccinations. An important finding is that in some patients some MBP-reactive T cell clonotypes, most likely present at low precursor frequencies at the time of the first vaccination, are upregulated after vaccination. It is possible that the anti-MBP repertoire in these patients changes in a dynamic way as seen in other studies (Goebels et al. 2000). To down-regulate all pathogenic T cell clones, these patients may need to be vaccinated several times.

Safety and regulatory issues. Although we did not observe any direct toxic effects of T cell vaccination in our pilot study, the current protocol involves long-term (3–4 months) in vitro culturing of T cells (in the presence of purified human brain antigens) which poses some concern about possible contamination with potential infectious agents. This could be avoided by the use of recombinant antigens.

Vaccine preparation. The current protocol involves isolation of myelin-reactive T cell lines and cloning of these lines. This is a laborious procedure that requires relatively large volumes of blood. This time-consuming, laborious protocol seriously hampers the widespread application of TCV.

Vaccine composition. The current T cell vaccine is composed of blood-derived autologous, activated, clonally expanded $CD4^+$ MBP-reactive T cell clones. There is however evidence suggesting that other anti-myelin T cell subsets (including anti-MOG and anti-PLP T cells) may also play an important role in the auto-immunity-mediated demyelination in MS. It may therefore be advantageous to incorporate these T cell populations in the vaccine to completely abolish pathogenic anti-myelin reactivity in individual patients. This however would significantly complicate the vaccination procedure. With the current protocol design it is almost impossible to incorporate T cell clones specific for three different myelin antigens.

On the basis of these limitations, we explored the possibility to use IL-2-expanded CD4 T lymphocytes from the cerebrospinal fluid (CSF) as vaccine. There is important evidence indicating that activated myelin-reactive T cells accumulate in the CSF of patients with MS, and low-dose IL-2 stimulation can be used to expand these cells from the CSF (Zhang et al. 1994). This approach has several advantages as compared to the original method. It is simpler, faster, requires less blood and can potentially be automated. On the other hand, the procedure does not lead to purified clones and the vaccine composition may therefore vary in time. Our preliminary data indicate that dominant clonotypes can be cultured from the CSF lymphocytes of MS patients. Five patients are currently involved in a pilot trial of CSF-based TCV. If this trial provides interesting data, a small double-blinded placebo-controlled study will be performed in early-relapsing-remitting MS patients with this TCV protocol. These studies and current trials in other centres in Jerusalem, Los Angeles, and Houston may provide further evidence for the usage of TCV and its potential effects in MS and will provide additional information on the most appropriate protocol to be used in future studies of TCV (see www.T-cellvaccination.org).

Acknowledgements. The help and assistance of the technical staff and other investigators of our laboratory is greatly appreciated. This research was funded by the Belgian Fonds voor Wetenschappelijk Onderzoek-Vlaanderen (FWO), the Vlaams Instituut voor Wetenschappelijk-Technologisch Onderzoek (IWT), the Belgian Charcot Foundation, the Wetenschappelijk Onderzoek Multiple Sclerose (WOMS) Foundation, the Fonds ter Bevordering van het Wetenschappelijk Onderzoek in het Dr. L. Willems-Instituut (FWI) and the Limburgs Universitair Centrum (LUC).

References

Ben-Nun A, Wekerle H, Cohen IR (1981) Vaccination against autoimmune encephalomyelitis with T-lymphocyte line cells reactive against myelin basic protein. Nature 292: 60–61

Cohen IR (1992) The cognitive paradigm and the immunological homunculus. Immunol Today 13: 490–494

Ffrench-Constant C (1994) Pathogenesis of multiple sclerosis. Lancet 343: 271–275

Goebels N, Hofstetter H, Schmidt S, Brunner C, Wekerle H, Hohlfeld R (2000) Repertoire dynamics of autoreactive T cells in multiple sclerosis patients and healthy subjects: epitope spreading versus clonal persistence. Brain 123: 508–518

Hafler DA, Kent SC, Pietrusewicz MJ, Khoury SJ, Weiner HL, Fukaura H (1997) Oral administration of myelin induces antigen-specific TGFβ1 secreting T cells in patients with multiple sclerosis. Ann NY Acad Sci 835: 120–131

Hemmer B, Vergelli M, Calabresi P, Huang T, McFarland HF, Martin R (1996) Cytokine phenotype of human autoreactive T cell clones specific for the immunodominant myelin basic protein peptide (83–99). J Neurosci Res 45: 852–862

Hemmer B, Vergelli M, Pinilla C, Houghten R, Martin R (1998) Probing degeneracy in T-cell recognition using peptide combinatorial libraries. Immunol Today 19: 163–168

Herkel J, Brunner S, Meyer zum Buschenfelde KH, Lohse AW (1997) Humoral mechanisms in T cell vaccination: induction and functional characterization of anti-lymphocytic autoantibodies. J Autoimmun 10: 137–146

Hermans G, Stinissen P, Hauben L, Van den Berg-Loonen E, Raus J, Zhang J (1997) Cytokine profile of myelin basic protein-reactive T cells in multiple sclerosis and healthy individuals. Ann Neurol 42: 18–27

Hermans G, Denzer U, Lohse A, Raus J, Stinissen P (1999) Cellular and humoral immune response against autoreactive T cells in multiple sclerosis patients after T cell vaccination. J Autoimmun 13: 233–246

Hermans G, Medaer R, Raus J, Stinissen P (2000) Myelin reactive T cells reappearing after T cell vaccination in multiple sclerosis: cytokine profile and depletion by additional immunizations. J Neuroimmunol 102: 79–84

Kos FJ, Engleman EG (1996) Immune regulation: a critical link between NK cells and CTLs. Immunol Today 17: 174–176

Kozovska MF, Yamamura T, Tabira T (1996) T-T cellular interaction between CD4⁻CD8⁻ regulatory T cells and T cell clones presenting TCR peptide. J Immunol 157: 1781–1790

Kumar V, Sercarz E (1998) Induction or protection from experimental autoimmune encephalomyelitis depends on the cytokine secretion profile of TCR peptide-specific regulatory CD4 T cells. J Immunol 161: 6585–6591

Lehmann PV, Sercarz EE, Forsthuber T, Dayan CM, Gammon G (1993) Determinant spreading and the dynamics of the autoimmune T-cell repertoire. Immunol Today 14: 203–208

Lider O, Reshef T, Beraud E, Ben-Nun A, Cohen IR (1988) Anti-idiotypic network induced by T cell vaccination against experimental autoimmune encephalomyelitis. Science 239: 181–183

Lohse AW, Mor F, Karin N, Cohen IR (1989) Control of experimental autoimmune encephalomyelitis by T cells responding to activated T cells. Science 244: 820–822

Lohse AW, Spahn TW, Wolfel T, Herkel J, Cohen IR, Meyer zum Buschenfelde KH (1993) Induction of the anti-ergotypic response. Int Immunol 5: 533–539

Medaer R, Stinissen P, Truyen L, Raus J, Zhang J (1995) Depletion of myelin-basic-protein autoreactive T cells by T cell vaccination: pilot trial in multiple sclerosis. Lancet 346: 807–808

Mor F, Reizis B, Cohen IR, Steinman L (1996) IL-2 and TNF receptors as targets of regulatory T-T interactions: isolation and characterization of cytokine receptor-reactive T cell lines in the Lewis rat. J Immunol 157: 4855–4861

Stinissen P, Zhang J, Medaer R, Vandevyver C, Raus J (1996) Vaccination with autoreactive T cells in multiple sclerosis: overview of immunological and clinical data. J Neurosci Res 45: 500–511.

Stinissen P, Raus J, Zhang J (1997) Autoimmune pathogenesis of multiple sclerosis: role of autoreactive T lymphocytes and new immunotherapeutic strategies. Crit Rev Immunol 17: 33–75

Stinissen P, Medaer R, Raus J (1998a) Myelin reactive T cells in the autoimmune pathogenesis of multiple sclerosis. Mult Scler 4: 203–211

Stinissen P, Zhang J, Vandevyver C, Hermans G, Raus J (1998b) γδ T cell responses to activated T cells in multiple sclerosis patients induced by T cell vaccination. J Neuroimmunol 87: 94–104

Stinissen P, Medaer R, Raus J (1998c) Preliminary data of an extended open label phase I study of T cell vaccination in multiple sclerosis. J Neuroimmunol 90: A564

Vandenbark AA, Chou YK, Whitham R, Mass M, Buenafe A, Liefeld D, Kavanagh D, Cooper S, Hashim GA, Offner H (1996) Treatment of multiple sclerosis with T cell receptor peptides: results of a double-blind pilot trial. Nat Med 2: 1109–1115

Waisman A, Ruiz PJ, Hirschberg DL, Gelman A, Oksenberg JR, Brocke S, Mor F, Cohen IR, Steinman L (1996) Suppressive vaccination with DNA encoding a variable region gene of the T-cell receptor prevents autoimmune encephalomyelitis and activates Th2 immunity. Nat Med 2: 899–905

Wucherpfennig KW, Strominger JL (1995) Molecular mimicry in T cell-mediated autoimmunity: viral peptides activate human T cell clones specific for myelin basic protein. Cell 80: 695–705

Zhang J, Medaer R, Stinissen P, Hafler D, Raus J (1993) MHC-restricted depletion of human myelin basic protein-reactive T cells by T cell vaccination. Science 261: 1451–1454

Zhang JW, Markovic S, Lacet B, Raus J, Weiner HL, Hafler DA (1994) Increased frequency of interleukin 2-responsive T cells specific for myelin basic protein and proteolipid protein in peripheral blood and cerebrospinal fluid of patients with multiple sclerosis. J Exp Med 179: 973–984.

Zhang J, Vandevyver C, Stinissen P, Raus J (1995) In vivo clonotypic regulation of human myelin basic protein-reactive T cells by T cell vaccination. J Immunol 155: 5868–5877

Plasmid-mediated delivery of antigens or biological response modifiers as means to suppress autoimmunity

Matthias von Herrath[1] and **Adrian Bot**[2,*]

[1]Department of Neuropharmacology and Immunology, Scripps Research Institute, La Jolla, and
[2]Department of Immunology, Alliance Pharmaceutical Corp., San Diego, California, U.S.A.

Introduction

The discovery of immunostimulatory motifs on bacterial DNA energized many laboratories, since it became evident that the associated Th1-driving ability is a positive feature, optimizing the quality of plasmid vectors as antiviral or antiallergic vaccines. In fact, the Th1 adjuvant activity of unmethylated CpG motifs can be even used to circumvent the inherently low and Th2-biased responsiveness of neonates. With all the advances during the last decade that promoted the initiation of clinical trials with DNA vaccines, a limiting factor was still the low magnitude of immunity.

In this circumstance, a potential application of plasmid vaccination towards suppressing Th1-controlled autoimmunity appears counterintuitive. Nevertheless, reports during the last five years described conditions when plasmid-mediated delivery of either self-antigens or biological response modifiers inhibited auto-immune processes. At the other end of the spectrum, a few studies documented aggravation of autoimmunity subsequent to exposure to plasmids or immuno-stimulatory motifs. Clearly, the main task to be accomplished is the definition of mechanisms of disease suppression by plasmid vaccination, together with the reasons of failure in certain conditions. This may set the stage for rational develop-ment of plasmid-based protocols of immunoprophylaxis or therapy of autoimmune diseases. In this chapter, we outline the preclinical experience with plasmid vectors in autoimmune diseases, potential mechanisms of activity, and future directions with roadblocks to be addressed.

* Author's address: Department of Immunology, Alliance Pharmaceutical Corp., 6175 Lusk Boulevard, San Diego, CA 92121, U.S.A.
E-mail: axb@allp.com

Potential pathways to down-regulate autoaggressive T cells

In autoimmune diseases, through various mechanisms, autoreactive lymphocytes escape the central and peripheral tolerance mechanisms. Depending on the disease or experimental model, genetic and environmental factors are involved to a different extent. For example, whereas NOD mice develop diabetes independently of exposure to environmental antigens, transgenic mice that express viral antigens in pancreas develop diabetes through cross-reaction with nonself-antigens. Designing strategies to suppress autoimmunity should take into consideration such points. For example, inducing antigen-dependent mediated cell death (AICD) by frequent inoculation of soluble antigen might by very difficult in individuals that are genetically defective in the Fas-mediated cell death pathway and/or signaling triggered by interleukin-2 (IL-2). As alternative approach, one may want to try switching the phenotype of the autoreactive T cells toward nonpathogenic or suppressor cells. A particular example would be the induction of anergy by virtue of activating the CTLA-4-dependent pathway (Chambers et al. 2001) that may be associated with the induction of IL-10-producing Tr1 cells (Stephens et al. 2001).

There are two tendencies that influence the direction of research in treating autoimmunity: first, a desire to achieve more specificity and optimal therapeutic index and secondly, in context of genomics advances and preclinical screening, to address both therapy and prophylaxis. Naturally, since the most specific markers for autoaggressive lymphocytes are the antigen-specific receptors themselves, a specific targeting strategy should take that into account. Thus, the interest in antigen-dependent immunotherapy or prophylaxis is maintained despite obvious setbacks in the past (Genain et al. 1996), caused by our limited understanding on how to control the outcome.

Plasmid-mediated delivery of self-antigens

Previous-generation antigen-based immunotherapeutics consisted in disease-associated peptides or proteins encompassing dominant epitopes. Due to low ability of such compounds to result in effective loading of major histocompatibility complex (MHC) II molecules, a discernable effect on immune response required large doses that were sometimes associated with unacceptable side effects. In addition, controlling the outcome in terms of the profile of immune response has been a very difficult task.

Use of plasmids to deliver self-antigens results in a peculiar pattern of lymphocyte exposure: minute amounts of antigen would continuously be produced by somatic cells and for a certain interval by few transfected antigen-presenting cells (APC) with the ability to migrate to local lymphoid organs. Would such pattern be compatible with AICD? Probably not, due to quantitative and "geographical" reasons, meaning only more localized antigen exposure to very limited amounts of antigen. Would, in turn, plasmid vaccination be compatible with CTLA-4-triggered anergy? What is the effect in this context of the powerful adjuvant ability of bacterial plasmid that enhances the expression of B7 co-stimulatory molecules on APC? While no one can yet exclude the employment of either one of the above mentioned pathways, alternative nonredundant mechanisms may still be triggered upon plasmid vaccination: for example, induction of antigen-specific regulatory cells (Th2, Th3, Tr1 or CD25$^+$) with the ability to migrate and expand in the target organ. The task would be to substantiate their induction and minimize, in parallel, an amplification of the autoaggressive pool. Can that be achieved by plasmid-mediated delivery? Preclinical data suggest yes, although the outcome is not invariably the same.

Basic immunological properties of bacterial DNA

There are three parameters of plasmid-based expression vectors that may interfere with the homeostasis of the immune system, responsible for self–nonself discrimination and regulation of response to antigens. First, the presence of immune stimulatory unmethylated CpG motifs in bacterial DNA (Krieg 1996, Tighe et al. 1998) is responsible for the Th1-promoting adjuvant activity. Secondly, the plasmid DNA itself acts like an antigen and may trigger the generation or enhancement of anti-DNA antibodies above pathological thresholds. Thirdly, the antigens expressed by plasmid-based vectors may cross-react to a certain extent with self-antigens. All these three properties, together with factors like route, frequency, and dose of inoculation, may be exploited with the aim of preventing or suppressing autoimmune conditions.

During the last few years, important advances were made regarding the mechanism by which unmethylated CpG motifs exert their immunomodulatory effects (Krieg et al. 1998). Exposure of APC to such motifs results in the activation of cytokine-producing pathways probably via engagement of Toll-like receptor 9 and activation of nuclear factor κB. It is generally accepted that a Th1-driving pattern of cytokines is triggered, although the route of plasmid inoculation may influence the outcome, depending perhaps on the local repertoire of APC. Most dramatically, coadministration of purified protein antigens and CpG motifs shifts the T cell profile from weak Th2 to strong Th1 associated even with induction of MHC I-restricted cytotoxic T lymphocytes (CTL) (Cho et al. 2000). At the first glance, in such circumstances the unavoidable presence of CpG motifs on most of the plasmid vectors employed would rather limit the use of this strategy, to enhancing antimicrobial responses or suppressing allergy.

Th1/Th2 paradigm: are plasmid expression vectors useful within the realm of inflammatory diseases?

Due to the presence of immunostimulatory motifs on bacterial DNA, Th1-mediated immune pathology as well as anti-DNA-antibody-mediated disease may be enhanced by genetic vaccination. Consequently, one may expect certain applications in the area of allergy and concerns regarding potential triggering or exacerbation of autoimmunity.

First, because the allergic phenomena are mediated by Th2 cells, the strong Th1-stimulatory activity of bacterial plasmid may be exploited with some benefits in this area. Earlier attempts to use DNA-based vaccines for suppressing allergic responses originated from the empirical observation that inoculation of plasmid expression vectors was associated with Th1 rather than Th2 immune responses. Induction of Th1 memory cells specific for allergens may down-regulate the subsequent priming of pathogenic Th2 cells, thus preventing allergic reactions. Hsu et al. (1996) reported that intramuscular inoculation of rats with a plasmid expressing a common allergen, Der p5 of the house dust mite, prevented the induction of specific immunoglobulin E (IgE) antibodies as well as asthma subsequent to aerosol sensitization. Using a different experimental system, an independent group showed similar results (Raz et al. 1996). Since the suppression of IgE antibodies occurred in a specific manner, namely, being restricted to the original antigen (Raz et al. 1996, Hsu et al. 1996), it is more probable that specific $CD8^+$ T cells primed by DNA vaccine are restimulated by protein or allergen. Moreover, this observation underlines the important role of the bacterial plasmid as expression vector for the allergen, a conclusion that is coherent with the inability of control plasmids to induce similar effects (Raz et al. 1996).

Due to the identification of bacterial CpG motifs that stimulate the innate immunity and Th1 responses, there has been a justified interest towards defining their therapeutic benefit in the context of allergy. A recent study, directly relevant for the potential of CpG oligodeoxynucleotides to suppress pathogenic Th2 responses, showed that coinoculation of oligonucleotides with allergen (*Schistosoma mansoni* eggs) prevented specific symptoms in a murine model for asthma (Kline et al. 1998). A significant clue regarding the role of immune stimulatory CpG motifs was provided by a study of the Th profile of immune response elicited by Bet v1, a major allergen of birch pollen, delivered as protein, via recombinant DNA with or without addition of CpG motifs (Hartl et al. 1999).

Together, this information indicates that: (1) DNA-based expression of allergen can prevent Th2 pathogenic responses; (2) CpG oligodeoxynucleotides may reproduce the effects of plasmids when administered together with the allergen; (3) thus, the amelioration of Th2 responses by using such compounds in previously sensitized organisms (Raz et al. 1996) is of great interest.

A recent report studied the immune response of mice immunized with a plasmid expressing the human thyrotropin receptor (hTSHR). The original aim of the study was to take advantage of DNA-based immunization strategy to raise antibodies against conformational epitopes of hTSHR, otherwise a difficult task to accomplish by inoculation of recombinant protein (Costagliola et al. 1998). Mice immunized with DNA developed hTSHR-specific antibodies that displayed blocking or activating function on the mouse receptor. Despite the lack of significant endocrine disturbances, the mice displayed massive lymphocytic infiltration in thyroid gland. In addition, plasmid vectors can be used to break the tolerance against tumor-associated self-antigens (Bronte et al. 2000).

A legitimate concern of DNA vaccines is the triggering of Th1-mediated organ-specific autoimmune diseases, since bacterial DNA has strong adjuvant activity. A first report examined this possibility and found that T cells specifically reactive to the myelin basic protein (MBP) exposed to bacterial DNA became pathogenic when adoptively transferred into experimental allergic encephalomyelitis (EAE) susceptible mice (Segal et al. 1997). However, the authors were able to induce an IL-12-dependent pathogenic phenotype of the MBP-specific T cells only by in vitro treatment with bacterial DNA or stimulatory motifs. Two subsequent studies by Tsunoda et al. (1998, 1999) showed that administration of plasmids expressing epitopes derived from the myelin proteolipid protein (PLP) in the context of allergic and infectious models of multiple sclerosis (MS) may actually result in exacerbation of disease. Of particular importance was the finding that plasmid vaccination in the context of Theiler's murine encephalomyelitis model of MS resulted in increased immune pathology without disabling the immune response against foreign viral antigen (Tsunoda et al. 1999). Anti-viral antibodies actually were substantiated, together with the production of gamma interferon (IFN-γ) and IL-6 cytokines. A recent, elegant study of Selmaj et al. (2000) discriminated for the first time conditions when plasmid vaccination leads to exacerbated versus ameliorated EAE disease in mice. Priming with a PLP-expressing vector resulted in a biphasic susceptibility profile: the early (10 weeks) stage when the mice developed exacerbated EAE upon injection of antigen plus adjuvant and a subsequent phase when mice were largely protected from aggravated disease due to down-regulation of Th1 and CTL not apparently associated with Th2 immunity. This study supports the concept that plasmid vaccination with self-antigen may elicit arms with opposing effects on disease, albeit of different persistency and potency. Controlling this phenomenon may allow a rationale design and use of plasmid vectors for suppressing autoimmune processes.

The preclinical experience in multiple sclerosis and rheumatoid arthritis models

An accumulating number of independent studies demonstrated that DNA vectors may be used to prevent the onset of autoimmunity in animal models (Table 1).

An initial report described the effect of immunization of Lewis rats with a plasmid expressing hsp65 on the induction of adjuvant arthritis (Ragno et al. 1997). Interestingly, despite the fact that rats preinoculated with plasmid displayed increased hsp65-specific antibody and T cell responses even after adjuvant

Table 1. Plasmid-mediated delivery of self-antigens in models of autoimmune diseases

Disease	Experimental model	Reference(s)
Rheumatoid arthritis	Adjuvant arthritis (hsp65 antigen)	Ragno et al. 1997
Multiple sclerosis	EAE (MBP)	Lobell et al. 1998, 1999; Weissert et al. 2000
	EAE (PLP)	Ruiz et al. 1999; Selmaj et al. 2000
	TMEV (VP 1-3)	Tolley et al. 1999
Autoimmune diabetes	RIP-NP-LCMV transgenic mice (InsB antigen)	Coon et al. 1999
	NOD mice (HSP60)	Quintana et al. 2000
	NOD mice (GAD65Fc + IL-4)	Tisch et al. 2001
	NOD mice (InsB)	Bot et al. 2001

injection, they were clinically protected against arthritis. Possibly, genetic immunization induced suppressor cells or, alternatively, directly down-regulated a subset of precursors of pathogenic T cells. Simultaneously, Ramshaw et al. (1997) suggested the application of this concept to other autoimmune diseases such as MS. A subsequent interesting report studied the effect of genetic immunization of Lewis rats on the susceptibility to EAE triggered by immunization with guinea pig MBP 68–85 peptide in complete Freund adjuvant (Lobell et al. 1998). The plasmid used for immunization expressed a similar peptide as well as a microbial motif responsible for the binding to Fc of IgG. Genetic immunization with this construct largely prevented the induction of EAE. However, there are three notable particularities of this study. First, the dose of plasmid used for immunization was approximately 10–100 times higher than the minimal doses that elicit immune responses. Secondly, there was no significant Th switch caused by genetic immunization in this model. Thirdly, the IgG binding ability of the expressed construct was required, suggesting that endogenous internalization via Fcγ receptors facilitated the suppressor effect of the peptide. This interesting and somewhat surprising result may be explained by one or both of the following mechanisms: FcγR-mediated targeting of antigen to professional APC (Zaghouani et al. 1993) followed by more effective antigen-induced T cell death and/or FcγR-mediated triggering of suppressor cytokines like IL-10 (Sutterwala et al. 1998) that might facilitate T cell anergy induction. Follow-up studies, while shedding some light on the mechanisms of suppression, certainly underlined an interesting characteristic of the EAE model, namely, the pleiotropic effect of IFN-γ. Thus, surprisingly, the elimination of immune stimulatory CpG motifs responsible for Th1 induction, from the MBP-expressing vector, abolished its suppressing effect (Lobell et al. 1999). Independently, another group showed that IFN-γ induction by noncoding bacterial DNA contributes to disease suppression (Boccaccio et al. 1999). These results are still at odds with a report demonstrating exacerbation of disease by preinjection of CpG motifs in SJL/J mice infected with Theiler's murine encephalomyelitis virus or inoculated with PLP peptides (Tsunoda et al. 1999). Such discrepancies stemming from mechanistic differences may reveal potentially important issues that have to be considered before employing large-scale antigen-based immune therapy via gene expression vectors: (1) the level of understanding the mechanism of disease in various clinical subpopulations; (2) the possibility of designing vectors that irrespective of the disease stage and variability of pathogenic factors are devoid of aggravating effects. Subsequent studies strengthened the concept of using plasmid vectors for suppressing EAE: for example, one of them suggested that DNA vaccination with an encephalitogenic PLP epitope suppressed the disease via anergy due to reduced costimulation, leading to decreased production of Th1 cytokines (including IFN-γ) in the brain (Ruiz et al. 1999). In the Lewis rat model, it was shown that DNA vaccination with one MBP epitope could not suppress the disease triggered by another MBP encephalitogenic epitope (Weissert et al. 2000), arguing against a bystander suppression mechanism. However, this may have been due to limited antigen exposure of regulatory cells subsequent to induction of disease by a different epitope, a situation reminiscent of single-epitope disease models.

A somewhat disturbing complexity in the mechanisms of immune-mediated pathology triggered by microbial infection with direct implications on therapeutic strategy has been recently revealed in a model of encephalomyelitis triggered by mouse infection with the Theiler's murine virus (Tolley et al. 1999). Thus, whereas DNA vaccination of mice – previous to infection – with VP2 and VP3 resulted in suppression of disease, immunization with the VP1 antigen of Theiler's virus resulted in significant aggravation. This important study pinpointed the need to understand the function of epitopes that are involved in immune-mediated pathology previous to designing antigen-based immune modulating regimens. However, interestingly, this observation may open an avenue for the prevention of microbe-induced immune-mediated pathology using rationally designed vaccines against protective but not pathogenic nonself-epitopes.

Thus, these recent studies led to surprising results because the plasmid-based vectors display intrinsic Th1 adjuvant properties as well as limited expression levels of antigens, making them on these theoretical grounds poor candidates for either Th2 switch or antigen-induced T cell death. Such studies suggested that rather by inducing Th2-regulatory cells, plasmid vaccines may act in MS models by inducing anergy, tolerance, or another form of negative regulation of auto-aggressive T cells.

The autoimmune diabetes experience: expansion of autoreactive T cells is not necessarily detrimental

Plasmid-mediated delivery of antigens associated with insulin-dependent diabetes mellitus (IDDM) may modify the reactivity of self-specific lymphocytes. An exploratory study showed induction or enhancement of anti-glutamic acid decarboxylase (GAD) humoral response upon vaccination with a GAD-expressing plasmid of BALB/c, C57BL/6 or NOD mice (Wiest-Landerburger et al. 1998). No effect on spontaneous disease in NOD mice has been reported by this study.

In contrast, in a transgenic model of autoimmune diabetes based on epitope mimicry, we showed that vaccination with DNA expressing the insulin B chain resulted in induction of regulatory CD4$^+$ T cells that migrated to the local lymph nodes and down-regulated the activity of anti-self CD8$^+$ T cells probably via IL-4 production (Coon et al. 1999). This was the first successful attempt to suppress IDDM by plasmid-mediated delivery of self-antigen. The effect was antigen-dependent since a plasmid expressing viral antigen (i.e., the nucleoprotein of lymphocytic choriomeningitis virus [LCMV], expressed in the transgenic islets) failed to suppress the autoimmune process. Most notably, repeated administration of plasmid after but not before triggering the disease by LCMV infection was more successful in preventing the development of full-blown diabetes.

We subsequently sought to extend these observations from the RIP-LCMV-NP transgenic mouse model to the NOD model of disease. Interestingly, a disease-suppressive effect was noted when an insulin B-(pInsB) but not a GAD 65-expressing plasmid (pGAD) was repeatedly administered during the preinfiltration and continuing with the prediabetic stage (1, 4, and 8 weeks) (Fig. 1A). In our model, the administration of control plasmid devoid of antigen reading frame

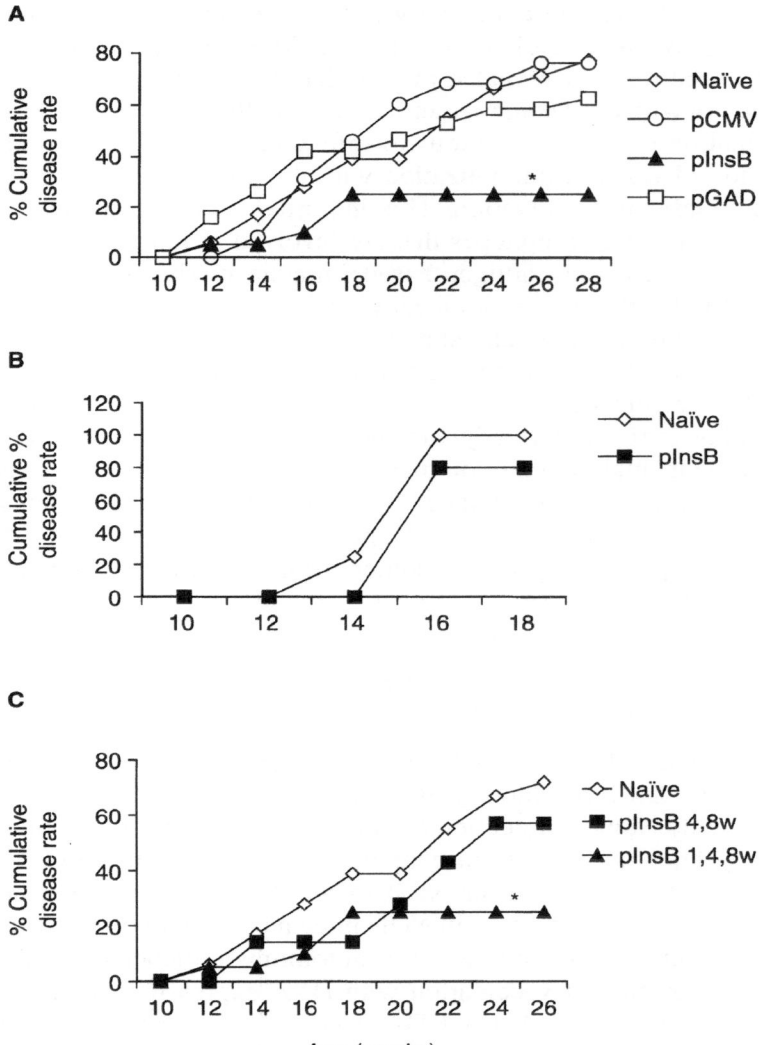

Fig. 1. A Female NOD mice were injected intramuscularly three times with plasmids expressing insulin B or GAD 65 antigens, or control plasmid, at the age of 1, 4, and 8 weeks. **B** Alternatively, IL-4null NOD mice were injected using the same protocol, with insulin B-expressing plasmid. **C** In a separate experiment, IL-4-competent female NOD mice were inoculated twice with insulin B-expressing plasmid, at the age of 4 and 8 weeks. The results were expressed as percentage of hyperglycaemic animals. *$P < 0.05$ (Fisher's exact test)

failed to modify the kinetics of disease (Fig. 1A) and had minimal influence on T cell profile (Bot et al. 2001). A peculiar finding in our model consisted in the lack of suppression of IDDM by pGAD treatment of female NOD mice (Fig. 1A). This is reminiscent of another recent study (Tisch et al. 2001) that showed effectiveness of GAD only when it was fused to the Fc segment of IgG and co-administered via a DNA expression vector together with IL-4 plasmid. In our study, characterization of the T cell profile in the spleens of female NOD mice immunized with pGAD showed expansion of Th1 cells reactive to dominant islet epitopes. In contrast, pInsB-vaccinated mice protected from disease showed a Th2-biased profile in the spleens (Bot et al. 2001). On the basis of all these considerations, we hypothesized that IL-4, a cytokine that is tightly associated with the Th2 response, may be critical in the protection from IDDM mediated by pInsB. As shown in Fig. 1B, indeed, in the absence of functional IL-4 genes, pInsB failed to prevent or suppress IDDM in female NOD mice.

The IL-4-dependent suppressive mechanism associated with the expansion of autoreactive but nonpathogenic T cells may be triggered by early, ectopic expression of self-antigen delivered via plasmid. This is suggested by the fact that neonatal DNA vaccination with foreign antigen triggered both Th1 and Th2 immunity, in contrast to adult DNA vaccination by intramuscular injection that generally results in induction of Th1 immunity (Bot et al. 1997). To test this hypothesis in the NOD model, we evaluated the effect of neonatal priming with pInsB on the development of IDDM. Strikingly, in the absence of neonatal priming, no substantial effect on the kinetics of disease was noted in female NOD mice (Fig. 1C). Together, the data in the pInsB-NOD mouse model suggest that protocols can be designed to achieve prophylaxis of IDDM with plasmid expression vectors.

Similar effects can be achieved with GAD-expressing plasmids; however, due to differential timing in the recruitment to the disease process, the immunization schedule and the precise coformulation should be different. The study of Tisch et al. (2001) correlates with our observations in three important aspects: first, it shows that GAD expressed by a plasmid is not effective in suppressing IDDM in NOD mice (unless fused to the Fc segment of and coadministered with IL-4); second, it demonstrates an antigen-specific effect of plasmid vaccination; and third, it supports an active suppressor mechanism via endogenous IL-4 production. The study of Quintana et al. (2000) carried out in NOD mice with a plasmid expressing HSP60 contrasts with Tisch et al. (2001) and Bot et al. (2001) since it shows a disease-suppressive effect triggered by CpG motifs, via modulation of HSP60 and p277-specific immunity. The plasmid expressing HSP60 inhibited the development of disease too, probably by shifting the nature of the T cell profile as indirectly suggested by antibody-isotype data (Quintana et al. 2000). In conclusion, three dominant antigens, GAD65, insulin B chain, and HSP60 may be used in the form of plasmid vaccines to suppress IDDM in animal models.

Mechanisms of action are still elusive

Three interesting dichotomies complicate the interpretation of mechanisms responsible for disease prevention and suppression by plasmid-mediated antigen delivery:

1. aggravation (Tsunoda et al. 1998, Selmaj et al. 2000) versus amelioration of disease (Ragno et al. 1997, Lobell et al. 1998, Coon et al. 1999, Quintana et al. 2000, Tisch et al. 2001, Bot et al. 2001) by plasmid vaccination;

Table 2. Potential disease-suppressive mechanisms elicited by plasmid-mediated delivery of self-antigens

Type of mechanism	Disease	Reference(s)	Evidence
Direct effect by anergy and/or deletion of pathogenic cells	EAE	Lobell et al. 1998	no Th1-to-Th2 shift
	EAE	Weissert et al. 2000	no bystander effect
Indirect effect by induction of regulatory cells	IDDM	Coon et al. 1999	protection from disease by adoptive transfer of CD4$^+$ T cells
	IDDM	Tisch et al. 2001; Bot et al. 2001	lack of protection of IL-4-null NOD mice
	RA	Ragno et al. 1997	enhanced immunity against disease-associated self-antigens

2. specificity (as suggested by most studies) versus lack of specificity (Boccaccio et al. 1999, Quintana et al. 2000) relative to encoded antigen;
3. regulatory and bystander versus targeted effect, as shown in Table 2.

In contrast to autoimmune diabetes and rheumatoid arthritis models, various plasmid vaccination protocols proved to worsen the disease in MS models. Tsunoda et al. (1998) demonstrated that PLP-expressing plasmids primed SJL/J mice for aggravated PLP-induced EAE disease. In contrast, Lobell et al. (1998) and Weissert et al. (2000) demonstrated suppression of disease in a Lewis rat-MBP model of MS. A recent study shed more light on this dichotomy, delineating conditions associated with aggravation or suppression of disease by plasmid vaccination with PLP (Selmaj et al. 2000). Short-term aggravating and long-term suppressing effects in this model suggested that long-lived regulatory T cells might have been induced. Alternatively but less likely due to quantitative reasons, AICD may have been triggered, preceded by transient expansion of pathogenic T cells. Nevertheless, simultaneous production of regulatory and nonpathogenic T cells and expansion of autoaggressive T cells subsequent to plasmid delivery may explain a series of apparently contradictory reports in the field.

One legitimate question is the double standard governing the outcome of plasmid-mediated delivery of self-antigens (mostly suppression of autoimmunity) versus foreign antigens, resulting in substantial induction of immune responses such as against viruses. Whatever the mechanism explaining aggravation versus amelioration of autoimmunity by plasmid vaccination, the intrinsic effect of immunostimulatory CpG motifs on bacterial DNA is puzzling. Conflicting reports demonstrated a disease-aggravating effect of bacterial DNA in mouse models of EAE (Tsunoda et al. 1999) and a rat model of MS, showing a dependency of the protection conferred by MBP-plasmid on the presence of CpG motifs (Lobell et al. 1999). A more recent study showed that nonexpressing plasmid can suppress autoimmune diabetes in NOD mice (Quintana et al. 2000), although subsequent studies in the same model failed to show similar effects (Tisch et al. 2001, Bot et al. 2001). An interplay between two categories of factors may explain these seemingly contradictory findings: first, the nature of plasmids used by different groups, with potentially distinct composition in immunostimulatory and immunosuppressor motifs; second, the diversity of disease models employed, with autoreactive T cells that may respond to distinct biological response modifiers (Boccaccio et al. 1999).

Earlier, the lack of Th1-to-Th2 shift combined with the requirement for CpG motifs in the protection conferred by plasmid vaccination with MBP against rat EAE (Lobell et al. 1998, 1999) argued against the involvement of Th2 regulatory T cells. A follow-up study brought up evidence against bystander suppression (Weissert et al. 2000), although the evidence presented may not be decisive due to peculiarities in the model employed. The facts in this particular model were concordant with the observations of Ruiz et al. (1999) of anergy induced by PLP-expressing plasmid, in EAE model. However, observations of Ragno et al. (1997) and Bot et al. (2001) showed an expansion of autoreactive T cells associated with protection from disease, in models of arthritis and IDDM, respectively. More compelling, Coon et al. (1999) showed that adoptive transfer of $CD4^+$ T cells from mice immunized with InsB-expressing plasmid transferred protection against IDDM. Such cells were able to limit the expansion of pathogenic $CD8^+$ CTL. In concordance with the suggestion that IL-4 may directly or indirectly be important for disease suppression by plasmid vaccination, both Tisch et al. (2001) and Bot et al. (2001) discovered that endogenous IL-4 expression was a prerequisite for the inhibition of IDDM by plasmids encoding GAD-Fc and InsB antigens, respectively. Whereas a suppressive effect of GAD was noted only when administered together with IL-4-expressing plasmid, the vaccination regimen with InsB needed to be started within the neonatal window, in order for the regimen to be effective. This is reminiscent of the earlier observation that neonatal DNA vaccination is more likely to trigger a non-Th1 (such as Th2) component (Bot et al. 1997).

Together, the studies carried out up to date unravel a complex network of factors determining the success of plasmid-mediated antigen immunoprophylaxis or therapy. Certain inoculation schedules and association with immunomodulatory factors may substantiate the protective effect. In addition, both the nature of antigen and the status and responsiveness of the specific T cell subset may be of paramount importance in determining the outcome. For example, a higher number of naïve low-affinity self-reactive T cells relative to differentiated, pathogenic cells may facilitate induction of anergy or regulatory cells. This can be achieved by early vaccination and substantiated by co-administration of biological response modifiers.

Plasmid-mediated transfer of biological response modifiers

Another strategy to control autoimmune diseases is by cytokine-mediated immune modulation. Administration of cytokines via plasmid-based expression vectors is not a very recent topics and has been first applied in the context of vaccination against microbes (Xiang and Ertl 1995).

An early report showed that monthly inoculation of plasmid expressing the transforming growth factor β into MLR/lpr/lpr mice, significantly delayed the onset and progression to systemic lupus erythematosus (Raz et al. 1995). Presumably, increased levels of systemic transforming growth factor β directly suppressed pathogenic T cells, slowing down the synthesis of IgG antibodies

specific for chromatin or Fc. In contrast, monthly inoculation of a plasmid expressing IL-2 had opposite effects, speeding up the onset of lupus in this experimental
model. Together, these results suggest that plasmid-mediated cytokine delivery
can be used for the purpose of immune modulation in autoimmune conditions.

More recently, a string of reports described successful modulation of EAE by
an indirect approach based on DNA vaccination, namely, raising immunity against
proinflammatory cytokines or chemokines. DNA vaccination with vectors expressing MIP-1α or MCP-1 – known to be maximally expressed in the brain after the
onset of disease – suppressed EAE (Youssef et al. 1998). Interestingly, although
vaccination with MIP-1β predisposed to aggravated disease, the authors proposed
that an immune response against proinflammatory C-C chemokines may have
explained the results. Subsequently, the authors showed that antibodies triggered
by chemokine-plasmid vaccination can transfer protection from disease, supporting their hypothesis (Yousseff et al. 2000). A different study in the same model
showed that DNA vaccination with a TNF-α expression vector raised anti-TNF-α
antibodies capable of inhibiting the EAE disease (Wildbaum and Karin 1999).
The authors subsequently extended this observation to a model of rheumatoid arthritis (Wildbaum et al. 2000a). A recent, elegant study of Wildbaum et al. (2000b)
showed that tolerance to FasL can be broken by DNA vaccination, with results on
suppressing EAE. Most interestingly, transfer of FasL binding antibodies at various
disease stages had differential effects on the outcome, revealing distinct roles for
Fas-mediated pathways during the pathogenesis. Early blocking of FasL led to
decreased production of TNF-α and suppression of disease, whereas late blocking
of FasL resulted in a failure to recover from acute disease.

It is interesting to notice, beyond the fact that some details of the mechanism
remain elusive, that such a strategy comprises the generation of antibody responses
by breakdown of tolerance to self-molecules via DNA vaccination.

Conclusions and future challenges

In view of the Th1-driving ability of CpG motifs, an intriguing application for
DNA vaccines is the field of autoimmune diseases. Clearly, more work is needed
to fully evaluate the potential practical value for such an application, supported
only by a few published studies. Efforts should be focused at characterizing the
conditions associated with DNA vaccination that promote autoimmunity versus
suppression or tolerance. This would eventually allow safer application of genetic
immunization in autoimmune diseases, as well as maximize their beneficial effects.
Early, prophylactic administration or employment of biological response modifiers
may optimize the therapeutic index of plasmid-based antigen delivery for suppression of autoimmunity.

Despite the recognized Th1-promoting adjuvant activity, plasmids have been
shown to successfully mediate local delivery of immunosuppressive cytokines
leading to the prevention of pathogenic Th1-mediated inflammation. That is still
another area that might prove fruitful from a practical point of view. In addition,
plasmids may be used to break the unresponsiveness to critical proinflammatory
molecules that contribute to the pathogenesis of autoimmune diseases.

In conclusion, before advancing to clinical trials, plasmid-based immunoprophylaxis and therapy faces two sets of milestones: one related to more profound understanding of the mechanisms of disease; and the other consisting in a better understanding of the potential of this method in the context of a particular disease.

References

Boccaccio GL, Mor F, Steinman L (1999) Non-coding plasmid DNA induces IFN-gamma in vivo and supresses autoimmune encephalomyelitis. Int Immunol 11: 289–296

Bot A, Antohi S, Bot S, Garcia-Sastre A, Bona C (1997) Induction of humoral and cellular immunity against influenza virus by immunization of newborn mice with a plasmid bearing a hemagglutinin gene. Int Immunol 9: 1641–1650

Bot A, Shearer M, Bot S, Avriette M, Garcia-Sastre A, White G, Woods C, Kennedy R, Bona C (2001) Induction of immunological memory in baboons primed with DNA vaccine as neonates. Vaccine 19: 1960–1967

Bot A, Smith D, Bot S, Hughes A, Wolfe T, Wang L, Woods C, von Herrath MG (2001) Plasmid vaccination with insulin B chain prevents autoimmune diabetes in NOD mice. J Immunol 167: 2950–2955

Bronte V, Appoloni E, Ronca R, Zamboni P, Overwijk WW, Surman L, Restifo NP, Zanovello P (2000) Genetic vaccination with self tyrosinase-related protein 2 caused melanoma eradication but not vitiligo. Cancer Res 15: 253–258

Chambers CA, Kuhns MS, Egen JG, Allison JP (2001) CTLA-4-mediated inhibition in regulation of T cell responses: mechanisms and manipulation in tumor immunotherapy. Annu Rev Immunol 19: 565–594

Cho HJ, Takabayashi K, Cheng PM, Nguyen MD, Corr M, Tuck S, Raz E (2000) Immunostimulatory DNA-based vaccines induce cytotoxic lymphocyte activity by a T-helper cell-independent mechanism. Nat Biotechnol 18: 509–514

Coon B, An LL, Whitton JL, von Herrath MG (1999) DNA immunization to prevent autoimmune diabetis. J Clin Invest 104: 189–194

Costagliola S, Rodien P, Many M-C, Ludgate M, Vassart G (1998) Genetic immunization against the human thyrotropin receptor causes thyroiditis and allows production of monoclonal antibodies recognizing the native receptor. J Immunol 160: 1458–1465

Genain CP, Abel K, Bemar N, Villinger F, Rosenberg DP, Linington C, Raine CS, Hauser SL (1996) Late complications of immune deviation therapy in a non-human primate. Science 274: 2054–2057

Hartl A, Kiesslich J, Weiss R, Bernhaupt A, Mostbock S, Scheiblhofer M, Ebner C, Ferreira F, Thalhamer J (1999) Immune responses after immunization with plasmid DNA encoding Bet v 1, the major allergen of birch pollen. J Allergy Clin Immunol 103: 107–113

Hsu CH, Chua KY, Tao MH, Lai YL, Wu HD, Huang SK, Hsieh KH (1996) Immunoprophylaxis of allergen-induced immunoglobulin E synthesis and airway hyperresponsiveness in vivo by genetic immunization. Nat Med 2: 540–544

Kline JN, Waldschmidt TJ, Businga TR, Lemish JE, Weinstock JV, Thorne PS, Krieg AM (1998) Modulation of airway inflamation by CpG oligodeoxynucleotides in a murine model of asthma. J Immunol 160: 2555–2559

Krieg AM (1996) Lymphocyte activation by CpG dinucleotide motifs in prokaryotic DNA. Trends Microbiol 4: 73–76

Krieg AM, Yi AK, Schorr J, Davis HL (1998) The role of CpG dinucleotides in DNA vaccines. Trends Microbiol 6: 23–27

Lobell A, Weissert R, Storch MK, Svanholm C, de Graaf KL, Lassmann H, Andersson R, Olsson T, Wigzell H (1998) Vaccination with DNA encoding an immunodominant myelin basic protein peptide targeted to Fc of immunoglobulin G suppresses experimental autoimmune encephalomyelitis. J Exp Med 187: 1543–1548

Lobell A, Weissert R, Eltayeb S, Svanholm C, Olsson T, Wigzell H (1999) Presence of CpG DNA and the local cytokine milieu determine the efficacy of supressive DNA vaccination in experimental autoimmune encephalomyelitis. J Immunol 163: 4754–4762

Quintana FJ, Rotem A, Carmi P, Cohen IR (2000) Vaccination with empty plasmid DNA or CpG oligode-oxynucleotides against diabetes in nonobese diabetic mice: modulation of spontaneous heat shock protein autoimmunity. J Immunol 165: 6148–6155

Ragno S, Colston MJ, Lowrie DB, Winrow VR, Blake DR, Tascon R (1997) Protection of rats from adjuvant arthritis by immunization with naked DNA encoding for mycobacterial heat shock protein 65. Arthritis Rheum 40: 277–283

Ramshaw IA, Fordham SA, Bernard CC, Maguire D, Cowden WB, Willenborg DO (1997) DNA vaccines for the treatment of autoimmune diseases. Immunol Cell Biol 75: 409–413

Raz E, Dudler J, Lotz M, Baird SM, Berry CC, Eisenberg RA, Carson DA (1995) Modulation of disease activity in murine systemic lupus erythematosus by cytokine gene delivery. Lupus 4: 286–292

Raz E, Tighe H, Sato Y, Corr M, Dudler JA, Roman M, Swain SL, Spiegelberg HL, Carson DA (1996) Preferential induction of a Th1 immune response and inhibition of specific IgE antibody formation by plasmid DNA immunization. Proc Natl Acad Sci USA 93: 5141–5145

Ruiz PJ, Garren H, Ruiz IU, Hirschberg DL, Nguyen LV, Karpuj MV, Cooper MT, Mitchell DJ, Fathman CG, Steinman L (1999) Suppressive immunization with DNA encoding a self-peptide prevents auto-immune disease: modulation of T cell costimulation. J Immunol 162: 3336–3341

Segal BM, Klinman DM, Shevach EM (1997) Microbial products induce autoimmune disease by an IL-12-dependent pathway. J Immunol 158: 5087–5090

Selmaj K, Kowal C, Walczak A, Nowicka J, Raine CS (2000) Naked DNA vaccination differentially modulates autoimmune processes in experimental autoimmune encephalomyelitis. J Neuroimmunol 111: 34–44

Stephens LA, Mottet C, Mason D, Powrie F (2001) Human CD4(+)CD25(+) thymocytes and peripheral T cells have immune suppressive activity in vitro. Eur J Immunol 31: 1247–1254

Sutterwala FS, Noel GJ, Salgame P, Mosser DM (1998) Reversal of proinflammatory responses by ligating the macrophage Fcγ receptor type I. J Exp Med 188: 217–222

Tighe H, Corr M, Roman M, Raz E (1998) Gene vaccination: plasmid DNA is more than just a blueprint. Immunol Today 19: 89–97

Tisch R, Wang B, Weaver DJ, Liu B, Bui T, Arthos J, Serreze DV (2001) Antigen-specific mediated suppression of beta cell autoimmunity by plasmid DNA vaccination. J Immunol 166: 2122–2132

Tolley ND, Tsunoda I, Fujinami RS (1999) DNA vaccination against Theiler's murine encephalomyelitis virus leads to alterations in demyelinating disease. J Virol 73: 993–1000

Tsunoda I, Kuang LQ, Tolley ND, Whitton JL, Fujinami RS (1998) Enhancement of experimental allergic encephalomyelitis (EAE) by immunization with myelin proteolipid protein (PLP) plasmid DNA. J Neuro-pathol Exp Neurol 57: 758–767

Tsunoda I, Tolley ND, Theil DJ, Whitton JL, Kobayashi H, Fujinami K (1999) Exacerbation of viral and autoimmune animal models for multiple sclerosis by bacterial DNA. Brain Pathol 9: 481–493

Weissert R, Lobell A, de Graaf KL, Eltayeb SY, Andersson R, Olsson M, Wigzell H (2000) Protective DNA vaccination against organ-specific autoimmunity is highly specific and discriminates between single amino acid substitutions in the peptide autoantigen. Proc Natl Acad Sci USA 97: 1689–1694

Wiest-Landenburger U, Fortnagel A, Richter W, Reimann J, Boehm B (1998) DNA vaccination with glutamic acid decarboxylase (GAD) generates strong humoral immune response in BALB/c, C57BL/6 and in diabetes prone NOD mice. Horm Metab Res 30: 605–609

Wildbaum G, Karin N (1999) Augumentation of natural immunity to a pro-inflamatory cytokine (TNF-alpha) by targeted DNA vaccine confers long-lasting resistance to experimental autoimmune encephalo-myelitis. Gene Ther 6: 1128–1138

Wildbaum G, Youssef S, Karin N (2000a) A targeted DNA vaccine augments the natural immune response against TNF-alpha and suppresses ongoing adjuvant arthritis. J Immunol 165: 5860–5866

Wildbaum G, Westermann J, Maor G, Karin N (2000b) A targeted DNA vaccine encoding Fas ligand defines its dual role in the regulation of experimental autoimmune encephalitis. J Clin Invest 106: 671–679

Youssef S, Wildbaum G, Maor G, Lanir N, Gour-Lavie A, Grabie N, Karin N (1998) Long lasting protec-tive immunity to experimental autoimmune encephalomyelitis following vaccination with naked DNA encoding C-C chemokines. J Immunol 161: 3870–3879

Youssef S, Maor G, Wildbaum G, Grabie N, Gour-Lavie A, Karin N (2000) C-C chemokine encoding DNA vaccines enhance breakdown of tolerance to their gene products and treat ongoing adjuvant arthritis. J Clin Invest 106: 361–371

Xiang ZQ, Ertl HC (1995) Manipulation of the immune response to a plasmid-encoded viral antigen by coinoculation with plasmids expressing cytokines. Immunity 2: 129–135

Zaghouani H, Steinman R, Nonacs R, Shah H, Gerhard W, Bona C (1993) Presentation of a viral T cell epitope expressed in the CDR3 region of a self immunoglobulin molecule. Science 259: 224–227

Intravenous immunoglobulins for the treatment of childhood autoimmune diseases

V. Wahn*

Klinikum Uckermark, Schwedt an der Oder, Federal Republic of Germany

Introduction

Over the last years it has become evident that intravenous immunoglobulins (IVIG) administered at high doses (HDIVIG) can have beneficial effects in autoimmune diseases. Most of the clinical information was obtained in patients with variants of immune thrombocytopenia (ITP). Further, most of the attempts to clarify the mode of action of HDIVIG have been made in ITP patients. Other inflammatory disorders pathogenetically unrelated to ITP also seem to respond to HDIVIG, and several authors have studied possible explanations for these effects. Table 1 summarizes biological effects supported by results from appropriate experiments. Further details can be found in comprehensive reviews (Ballow 1997, Kazatchkine and Kaveri 2001). This review focusses on mechanisms of HDIVIG in both ITP and other disorders.

Release of platelets from reticuloendothelial system

Schmidt et al. (1984) labelled autologous platelets with radioactive chromium in one child with ITP in order to study the effects of HDIVIG. HDIVIG caused a dilution of radioactive platelets indicating a release of unlabelled platelets from the reticuloendothelial system. This observation has never been extended to studies of a larger number of patients.

Influence on platelet-associated immunoglobulin G

Immunoglobulin G (IgG) can bind to platelets via the $F(ab')_2$ fragment if platelet-specific antibodies are present. Further, binding can occur via the Fc fragment if

* Author's address: Klinikum Uckermark, Auguststrasse 23, 16303 Schwedt an der Oder, Federal Republic of Germany.
E-mail: v.wahn@klinikum-uckermark.de

Table 1. Immunomodulatory effects of HDIVIG in ITP and other autoimmune disorders

---

Release of platelets from liver and spleen
Influence on platelet-associated IgG
   Reduction of synthesis
   Reduction of binding to platelets
Increased elimination of circulating and tissue-bound immune complexes
Blockade of Fc receptors by:
   IgG-Fc
   IgG antibodies to low-affinity FcR (CD16)
   Nonspecifically coated erythrocytes
   Erythrocytes coated with anti-D (rhesus D-positive individuals)
   Stimulation of inhibitory Fc receptor FcγRIIb
Saturation of neonatal Fc receptor
Inhibition of cell adhesion by natural RGD antibodies
Influences on complement system
Inhibition of (auto)antigen presentation and recognition of:
   Soluble membrane molecules
   Antibodies to important membrane molecules
Interference with idiotype-antiidiotype network
Neutralization of cytokines
Neutralization of superantigens
Influences on apoptosis
   Blockade of CD95
   Induction of apoptosis in lymphocytes and monocytes via the Fas pathway

---

immune complexes consisting of IgG and a viral antigen are present. Platelets express receptors for IgG Fc. Tsubakio et al. (1983) described that HDIVIG reduced the extent of antiplatelet antibody formation, while Winiarski et al. (1983) demonstrated competitive inhibition of autoantibody binding to platelets by HDIVIG. Free platelet autoantibodies increased following administration of HDIVIG.

Accelerated elimination of circulating and tissue-bound immune complexes

Imbach and Jungi (1983) discussed an accelerated elimination of circulating and tissue-bound immune complexes as a possible HDIVIG mechanism. Experimental evidence for this hypothesis comes from studies in lupus patients who following IVIG therapy showed decreasing immune complex titers (Lin and Racis 1986). Puddu et al. (1996) investigated skin biopsies from lupus patients and documented solubilization of immune complex in skin biopsies following HDIVIG.

Blockade of Fc receptors

Most authors consider the interaction with Fc receptors (FcR) the major mode of action of HDIVIG (Fig. 1). The overall effect can be subdivided into several individual mechanisms. When administered at high doses, IgG can bind with its

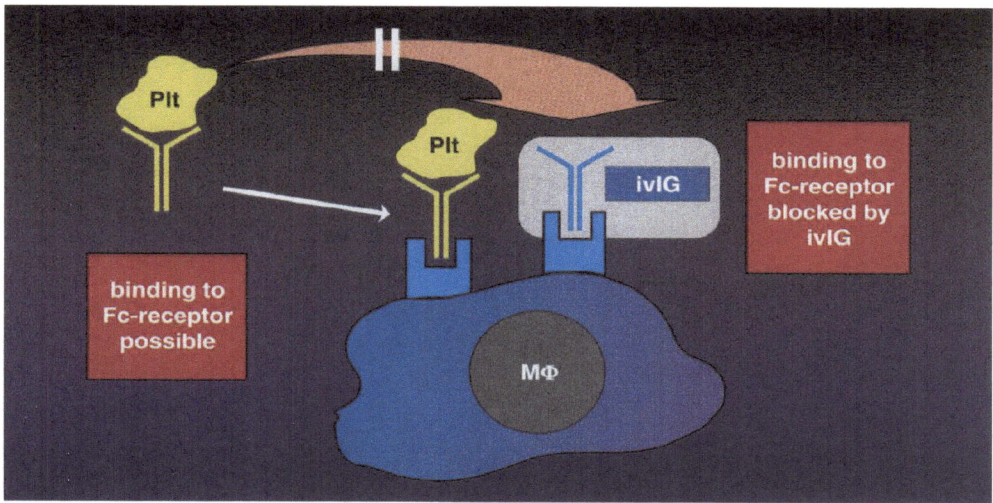

Fig. 1. Under normal circumstances antibody-coated platelets bind to Fc receptors (CD16, CD32, CD64) of reticuloendothelial cells and are eliminated via this route. HDIVIG blocks these receptors, of which CD16 seems to be the most important one

Fc portion to FcR. Evidence comes from experiments showing that the clearance of radioactively labelled autologous erythrocytes coated with anti-D antibody (these are also eliminated via interaction with Fc receptors) is markedly reduced in the presence of HDIVIG (Fehr et al. 1982). Final proof of principle comes from the publication of Debré et al. (1993), who showed that purified IgG Fc fragments induced remission in a high proportion of children with ITP.

Templeton et al. (1985) found that Fc receptors can be blocked not only by Fc fragments of IgG but also by autoantibodies directed against the low-affinity IgG Fc receptor CD16. Such antibody activity was shown in IVIG preparations. This mechanism may be relevant in vivo because Clarkson et al. (1986) were able to show that in an adult with ITP an increase of platelets could be achieved by parenteral administration of a monoclonal antibody to CD16.

Salama et al. (1983) focussed their work on another aspect. They showed that erythrocytes can be coated by IVIG nonspecifically but also specifically by irregular anti-D antibodies present at low titers in some preparations. IgG-coated erythrocytes compete with IgG-coated platelets for Fc receptors (Fig. 2). On the basis of this concept, ITP treatment with anti-D was developed where a few milligrams of specific anti-D immunoglobulin in rhesus-positive patients had the same effect as many grams of a polyvalent preparation.

Modulation of inhibitory Fc receptor

Monocytes express both stimulatory and inhibitory Fc receptors on their surface. Such inhibitory Fc receptors have been demonstrated in experimental animals

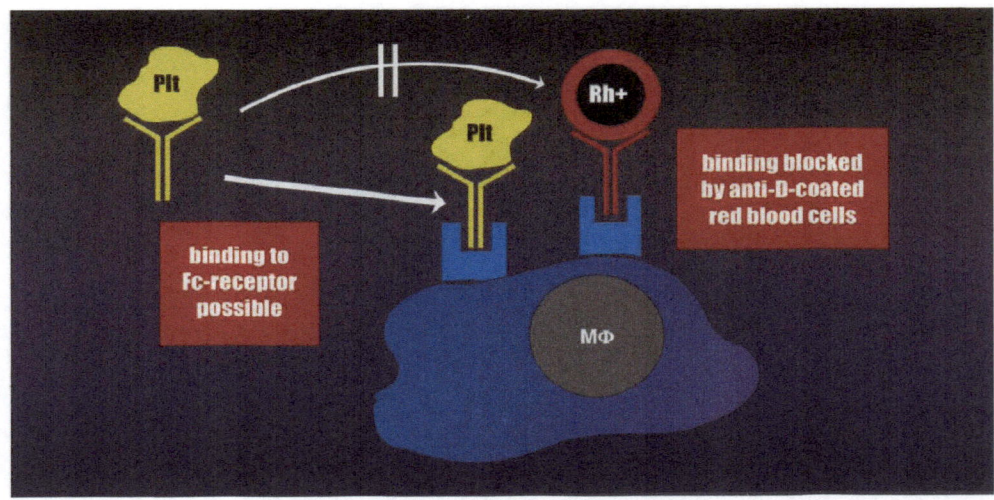

Fig. 2. Rhesus-positive erythrocytes coated with anti-D can compete with antibody-coated platelets for the binding sites at cellular Fc receptors

and humans. Samuelsson et al. (2001) were able to show in an animal model that IVIG induces the expression of an inhibitory FcγRIIB able to induce intracellular signalling which makes the monocyte unable to take up antibody-coated platelets (Fig. 3).

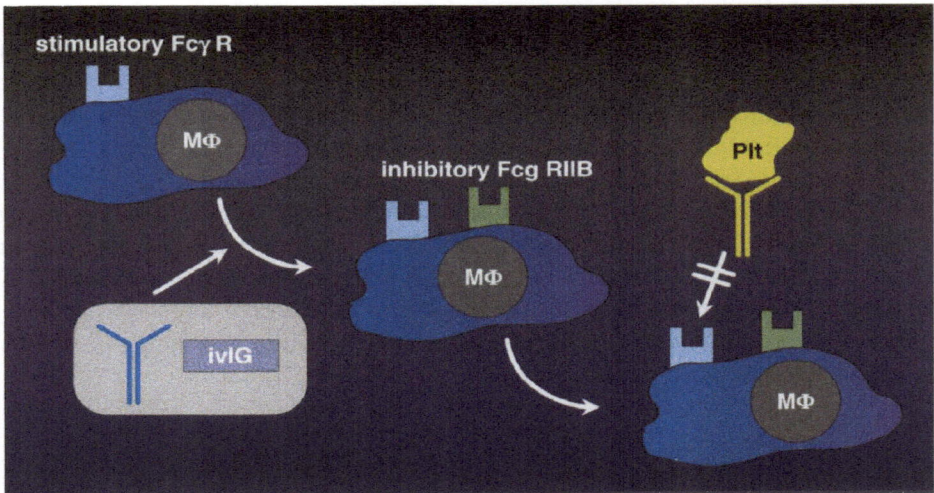

Fig. 3. IVIG stimulates the expression of an inhibitory Fc receptor, FcγRIIB, on monocytes and seems to trigger signals that render the stimulatory FcγR unable to take up antibody-coated platelets. Thus, these platelets remain in the circulation. From Samuelsson et al. (2001)

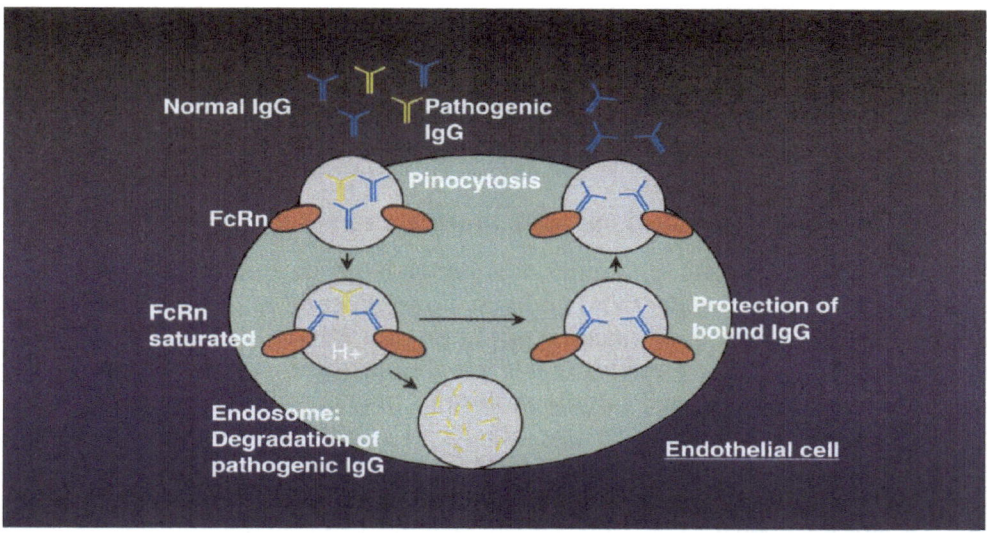

Fig. 4. IgG can be taken up to the endosomal compartment by endothelial cells by pinocytosis and binds to FcRn, the "neonatal" Fc receptor. This binding protects IgG from digestion in acidic environment. HDIVIG causes a competition of protective (blue) and pathogenic (yellow) immunoglobulins for FcRn. Pathogenic antibodies are shifted towards the low-pH compartment and are digested. From Yu and Lennon (1990)

Saturation of neonatal Fc receptor

Immunoglobulin levels in blood are regulated by several mechanisms. A new interesting aspect has been highlighted by Yu und Lennon (1999): Immunoglobulins taken up intracellularly in endosomes are digested in the acidic environment if not bound to the endosomal neonatal FcR. Binding protects against digestion. When IVIG is given at high doses, it prevents binding of pathogenic autoantibodies to FcRn and induces their shift towards the acidic compartment with subsequent hydrolysis (Fig. 4).

Inhibition of cellular adhesion by natural RGD antibodies

Vassilev et al. (1999) demonstrated antibodies in IVIG directed against the Arg-Gly-Asp sequence (so-called RGD sequence) which are part of the binding sites of certain surface molecules and extracellular matrix proteins, for example, in ligands for $\beta 1$-, $\beta 3$-, and $\beta 5$-integrins. IVIG activity depends on the $F(ab')_2$ fragments and is directed not only against RGD but also against fibronectin. Several cellular interactions of platelets and B cells depending on fibronectin are inhibited by anti-RGD $F(ab')_2$.

Influences on complement system

Some hemocytopenias pathogenetically involve the complement system. In certain animal models, IgM-coated erythrocytes are eliminated exclusively under participation of complement. HDIVIG markedly slowed down the elimination of such erythrocytes (Basta et al. 1989). Further, C3b inactivation in IgG immune complexes at least in vitro is accelerated due to the combined action of factors I and H (Lutz et al. 1996). Complement following the administration of HDIVIG becomes activated in vivo (Mollnes et al. 1998).

Modulation of (auto)antigen presentation and recognition

The synthesis of specific autoantibodies depends on the interaction of antigen-presenting cells and T cells. IVIG contains non-IgG soluble molecules which are probably released during the manufacturing process (Blaszyk et al. 1993). CD4 or major histocompatibility complex (MHC) II are intimately involved in the antigen recognition process and such soluble molecules may possibly interfere with it.

IVIG contains antibodies to important cell surface molecules. Kaveri et al. (1996) described antibodies against MHC I which were able to interfere with the function of cytotoxic T cells. These antibodies could be removed from the MHC I binding site by a MHC I peptide which resulted in normalization of cytotoxic-T-lymphocyte activity. Further autoantibodies in IVIG have been described against the T cell receptor (Marchalonis et al. 1992), MHC II (Moinier et al. 1987), or CD5 (Vassilev et al. 1993). Other regulatory mechanisms are discussed in a comprehensive review by Schiff (1994).

Interference with the idiotype-antiidiotype network

During the process of a B cell response to an antigen, antibodies are generated expressing a so-called idiotype in the hypervariable region consisting of a well-defined cross-reactive and a non-cross-reactive private region (Nydegger et al. 1984). An idiotype can induce an antiidiotypic immune response. Such antiidiotypic antibodies have been found in IVIG capable of binding to the idiotype of an autoantibody who, in turn, prevent its binding to the target autoantigen. Table 2

Table 2. Antiidiotypic antibodies in IVIG

Autoantibody	Titer [a]	
	before chromatography	after chromatography
Anti-F VIII F(ab')$_2$	0.8 BU/mg	38.08 BU/mg
Antithyroglobulin F(ab')$_2$	1.26 AU/mg	18.20 AU/mg
Anti-DNA-IgG	0.31 AU/mg	10.80 AU/mg
Anti-intrinsic factor IgG	3.26 AU/mg	4.32 AU/mg
Antineutrophil cytoplasmic antibody	1.12 AU/µg	3.4 AU/µg
Anti-retinal Ag S F(ab')$_2$	1.08 AU/mg	6.17 AU/mg

[a] The titer depends on the degree of enrichment following affinity chromatography (from Kaveri et al. 1991). BU, Bethesda units; AU, arbitrary units

summarizes some titers of such antiidiotypic antibodies. Commercial IVIG preparations contain IgG dimers and some evidence exists that these dimers are nothing but complexes of regular and antiidiotypic antibodies (Tankersley et al. 1988).

Silvestris et al. (1996) purified such antiidiotypic antibodies from commercial IVIG against double-stranded DNA autoantibodies and subsequently treated patients with systemic lupus erythematosus. In a few patients suffering from lupus nephritis they observed reduction of proteinuria, reduction of anti-DNA antibodies, and modulation of interleukin-6 (IL-6) and tumor necrosis factor alpha (TNF-α).

Neutralization of cytokines

The mechanisms illustrated so far do not sufficiently explain the efficacy of HD-IVIG even in the absence of demonstrable autoantibodies. Interference with the function of proinflammatory cytokines may be a reasonable explanation. In one study, antibodies to IL-1 and TNF were found in IVIG preparations (Andersson et al. 1990, Abe et al. 1994), while other authors showed downregulation of such cytokines (Shimozato et al. 1991). Both mechanisms in concert may result in a decreased ability of proinflammatory cytokines to support the inflammatory process. It was further shown in vitro that IVIG was capable of releasing the IL-1 receptor antagonist (IL-1RA) from monocytes. IL-1RA competes with IL-1 for the receptor binding site (Arend and Leung 1994, Mouthon et al. 1996). Aukrust et al. (1994) studied patients with hypogammaglobulinemia in vivo following the administration of immunoglobulins. Besides an increase of IL-1RA, they observed an increase of soluble TNF receptors. In later studies an increase of IL-1RA and neutralizing antibodies against IL-1α and sIL1-RII was observed accompanied by a decrease of IL-1α, IL-1β and sIL-1RI (Aukrust et al. 1999).

Neutralization of superantigens

Superantigens in contrast to regular antigens are not processed by antigen-presenting cells. On the basis of their dual affinity to both MHC II and relatively invariant T cell receptor sequences, they are capable of stimulating whole T cell families expressing certain Vβ chains (Fig. 5). The consequences of such massive T cell activation can be observed in certain human diseases where some evidence exists regarding a pathogenetic role for superantigens, like Kawasaki syndrome or toxic-shock syndrome. In IVIG, antibodies against such superantigens have been found which neutralize superantigen function (Takei et al. 1993).

Influence on apoptosis

Apoptosis is a multistep process initiated by interaction of CD95 with its ligand CD95L which finally results in programmed cell death. Apoptosis does not require enzymes released from cytotoxic granules used by cytotoxic T cells or NK cells. With respect to inflammatory or autoimmune disorders, apoptosis may be relevant

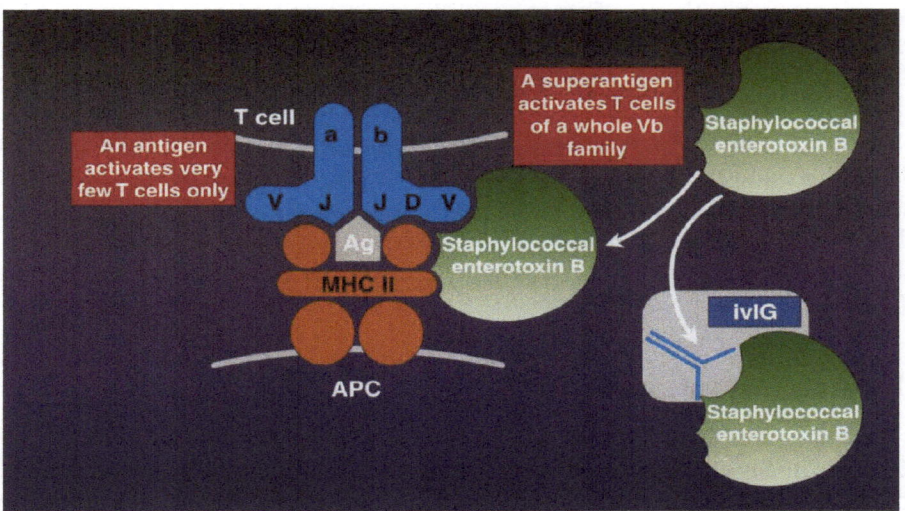

Fig. 5. In certain diseases like Kawasaki syndrome or toxic-shock syndrome, superantigens play an important role in the pathogenesis. IVIG is able to neutralize such superantigens and thus prevents massive T cell activation. From Takei et al. (1993)

because the deletion of pathogenic T cells may protect from autoimmunity. In contrast, persistence of such T cells may predispose to autoimmunity as shown in the autoimmune lymphoproliferative syndrome.

With regard to apoptosis, IVIG was studied in two respects. Prasad et al. (1998) used several cell lines in vitro and showed that IVIG contains anti-CD95 antibodies which can be enriched in titers 100-fold by affinity chromatography. Such antibodies induce apoptosis upon binding to CD95. The authors speculated that IgG in this way may participate in the control of cell proliferation.

A different situation is observed in toxic epidermal necrolysis (Lyell syndrome). In this disease patients develop apoptosis of keratinocytes of the skin which results in the separation of the dermal-epidermal junction zone and development of blisters. Viard et al. (1999) treated 10 Lyell patients with HDIVIG and found that it markedly reduced keratinocyte apoptosis. So we have evidence that IVIG exerts both stimulatory and inhibitory effects on CD95.

Summary

For many effects of IVIG experimental evidence has been obtained. The contribution of individual mechanisms may depend on the disease, i.e., in hematological disorders Fc receptor modulation may be most important, while it may be cytokine modulation in inflammatory disorders. Our knowledge about mechanisms may contribute to the development of useful hypotheses which will then have to be tested in clinical settings. These clinical studies will finally define the potential and the limitations of HDIVIG in autoimmune diseases.

References

Abe Y, Horiuchi A, Masazumi M, Kimura S (1994) Anti-cytokine nature of natural human immunoglobulin: one possible mechanism of the clinical effect of intravenous immunoglobulin therapy. Immunol Rev 139: 5–19

Andersson JP, Andersson UG (1990) Human intravenous immunoglobulin modulates monokine production in vitro. Immunology 71: 372–376

Arend WP, Leung DYM (1994) IgG induction of IL-1 receptor antagonist production by human monocytes. Immunol Rev 139: 71–78

Ashkenazi A, Dixit VM (1998) Death receptors: signaling and modulation. Science 281: 1305–1308

Aukrust P, Froland SS, Liabakk NB, Müller F, Nordoy I, Haug C, Espevik T (1994) Release of cytokines, soluble cytokine receptors, and interleukin-1 receptor antagonist after intravenous immunoglobulin administration in vivo. Blood 84: 2136–2143

Aukrust P, Müller F, Svensson M, Nordoy I, Bendtzen K, Froland SS (1999) Administration of intravenous immunoglobulin (IVIG) in vivo: down-regulatory effects on the IL-1 system. Clin Exp Immunol 115: 136–143

Ballow M (1997) Mechanisms of action of intravenous immune serum globulin in autoimmune and inflammatory diseases. J Allergy Clin Immunol 100: 151–157

Basta M, Langlois PF, Marques M, Frank MM, Fries LF (1989) High-dose intravenous immunoglobulin modifies complement-mediated clearance in vivo. Blood 74: 326–333

Blaszyk R, Westhoff U, Grosse-Wilde H (1993) Soluble CD4, CD8, and HLA molecules in commercial immunoglobulin preparations. Lancet 341: 789–790

Clarkson SB, Bussel JB, Kimberly RP, Valinsky JE, Nachman RL, Unkeless JC (1986) Treatment of refractory immune thrombocytopenic purpura with an anti-Fcγ-receptor antibody. N Engl J Med 314: 1236–1239

Debré M, Bonnet MC, Fridman WH, Carosella E, Philippe N, Reinert P, Vilmer E (1993) Infusion of Fcγ fragments for treatment of children with acute immune thrombocytopenic purpura. Lancet 342: 945–949

Fehr J, Hofmann V, Kappeler U (1982) Transient reversal of thrombocytopenia by high-dose intravenous gammaglobulin. N Engl J Med 306: 1254–1258

Imbach P, Jungi TW (1983) Possible mechanisms of intravenous immunoglobulin treatment in childhood idiopathic thrombocytopenic purpura (ITP). Blut 46: 117–124

Kaveri S, Dietrich G, Hurez V, Kazatchkine MD (1991) Intravenous immunoglobulins (IVIG) in the treatment of autoimmune diseases. Clin Exp Immunol 86: 192–198

Kaveri S, Vassilev T, Hurez V, Lengagne R, Lefranc C, Cot S, Pouletty P, Glotz D, Kazatchkine MD (1996) Antibodies to a conserved region of HLA class I molecules, capable of modulating CD8 T-cell-mediated function, are present in pooled normal immunoglobulin for therapeutic use. J Clin Invest 97: 865–869

Kazatchkine MD, Kaveri SV (2001) Immunomodulation of autoimmune and inflammatory diseases with intravenous immune globulin. N Engl J Med 345: 747–755

Lin RY, Racis SP (1986) In vivo reduction of circulating C1q binding immune complexes by intravenous gammaglobulin administration. Int Arch Allergy Appl Immunol 79: 286–290

Lutz HU, Stammler P, Jelezarova E, Nater M, Späth PJ (1996) High doses of immunoglobulin G attenuate immune aggregate-mediated complement activation by enhancing physiologic cleavage of C3b in C3b(n)-IgG complexes. Blood 88: 184–193

Marchalonis JJ, Kaymaz H, Dedeoglu F, Schluter SF, Yocum DE, Edmundson AB (1992). Human auto-antibodies reactive with synthetic autoantigens from T-cell receptor beta chain. Proc Natl Acad Sci USA 89: 3325–3329

Moynier M, Cosso B, Brochier J, Clot J (1987) Identification of class II HLA alloantibodies in placenta-eluted gamma-globulin used for treating rheumatoid arthritis. Arthritis Rheum 30: 375–381

Mouthon L, Kaveri SV, Spalter SH, Lacroix-Desmazes S, Lefranc C, Desai R, Kazatchkine MD (1996) Mechanism of action of intravenous immune globulin in immune-mediated diseases. Clin Exp Immunol 104 Suppl 1: 3–9

Nydegger UE, Blaser K, Hässig A (1984) Antiidiotype immunosuppression and its treatment with human immunoglobulin preparations. Vox Sang 47: 92–95

Prasad NKA, Papoff G, Zeuner A, Bonnin E, Kazatchkine MD, Ruberti G, Kaveri SV (1998) Therapeutic preparations of normal polyspecific IgG (IVIG) induce apoptosis in human lymphocytes and monocytes: a novel mechanism of action of IVIG involving the Fas apoptotic pathway. J Immunol 161: 3781–3790

Puddu P, de Pita O, Ruffelli M, Bellucci AM, Girardelli CR, Galeazzi M, Marcolongo R (1996) Intravenous immunoglobulin therapy: modification of the immunofluorescence pattern in the skin of six patients with systemic lupus erythematosus. Arthritis Rheum 39: 704–705

Salama A, Müller-Eckhardt C, Kiefel V (1983) Effect of intravenous immunoglobulin in immune thrombocytopenia. Lancet II: 193–195

Samuelsson A, Towers TL, Ravetch JV (2001) Anti-inflammatory activity of IVIG mediated through the inhibitory Fc receptor. Science 291: 484–486

Schiff RI (1994) Intravenous gammaglobulin 2: pharmacology, clinical uses and mechanisms of action. Pediatr Allergy Immunol 5: 127–156

Schmidt KG, Rasmussen JW, Diederichsen H, Ulrich M (1984) Release of platelets into the circulation induced by gamma globulin treatment in a case of idiopathic thrombocytopenic purpura. Blut 48: 27–31

Shimozato T, Iwata M, Kawada H, Tamura N (1991) Human immunoglobulin preparation for intravenous use induces elevation of cellular cyclic adenosine 3′:5′-monophosphate levels, resulting in suppression of tumor necrosis factor alpha and interleukin-1 production. Immunology 72: 497–501

Silvestris F, D'Amore O, Cafforio P, Savino L, Dammacco F (1996) Intravenous immune globulin therapy of lupus nephritis: use of pathogenic anti-DNA-reactive IgG. Clin Exp Immunol 104 Suppl 1: 91–97

Takei S, Arora YK, Walker SM (1993) Intravenous immunoglobulin contains specific antibodies inhibitory to activation of T cells by staphylococcal toxin superantigens. J Clin Invest 91: 602–607

Tankersley DL, Preston MS, Finlayson JS (1988) Immunoglobulin G dimer: an idiotype-anti-idiotype complex. Mol Immunol 25: 41–48

Templeton JG, Cocker JE, Crawford RJ, Forwell MA, Sandilands GP (1985) Fc gamma-receptor blocking antibodies in hyperimmune and normal pooled gammaglobulin. Lancet I: 1337

Tsubakio T, Kurata Y, Katagiri S, Kanakura Y, Tamaki T, Kuyama J, Kanayama Y, Yonezawa T, Tarui S (1983) Alteration of T cell subsets and immunoglobulin synthesis in vitro during high-dose γ-globulin therapy in patients with idiopathic thrombocytopenic purpura. Clin Exp Immunol 53: 697–702

Vassilev T, Gelin C, Kaveri SV, Zilber MT, Boumsell L, Kazatchkine MD (1993) Antibodies to the CD5 molecule in normal human immunoglobulins for therapeutic use. Clin Exp Immunol 92: 369–372

Vassilev TL, Kazatchkine MD, van Huyen JPD, Mekrache M, Bonnin E, Mani JC, Lecroubier C, Korinth D, Baruch D, Schriever F, Kaveri SV (1999) Inhibition of cell adhesion by antibodies to Arg-Gly-Asp (RGD) in normal immunoglobulin for therapeutic use (intravenous immunoglobulin, IVIG). Blood 93: 3624–3631

Viard I, Wehrli P, Bullani R, Schneider P, Holler N, Salomon D, Hunziker T, Saurat JH, Tschopp J, French LE (1998) Inhibition of toxic epidermal necrolysis by blockade of CD95 with human intravenous immunoglobulin. Science 282: 490–493

Winiarski J, Kreuger A, Ejderhamn J, Holm G (1983) High dose intravenous IgG reduces platelet associated immunoglobulins and complement in idiopathic thrombocytopenic purpura. Scand J Hematol 31: 342–348

Yu Z, Lennon VA (1999) Mechanism of intravenous immune globulin therapy in antibody-mediated autoimmune diseases. N Engl J Med 340: 227–228

SpringerMedicine

Michael Hertl (ed.)

Autoimmune Diseases of the Skin

Pathogenesis, Diagnosis, Management

2001. XVII, 373 pages. Numerous figures, partly in colour.
Hardcover **EUR 49,–**
(Recommended retail price)
Net-price subject to local VAT.
ISBN 3-211-83598-9

Cutaneous autoimmune diseases of the skin remain an enigma for many clinicians and scientists who are not familiar with these mostly severe and chronic diseases. The book presented provides an overview and the latest information on the broad spectrum of cutaneous autoimmune disorders for clinicians, scientists and practitioners in dermatology, medicine, rheumatology, ENT, pediatrics and ophthalmology.

The book is unique since it presents the state-of-the-art knowledge on pathophysiology, clinical diagnosis and management of these disorders provided by the world experts in the field. The primary intention is to broaden the understanding of the pathophysiology of cutaneous autoimmune disorders and to provide a practical guide to how to identify and handle these conditions. The book is illustrated with many tables, illustrative figures and clinical color photographs.

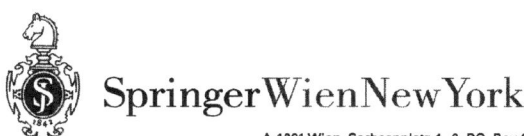

SpringerWienNewYork

A-1201 Wien, Sachsenplatz 4–6, P.O. Box 89, Fax +43.1.330 24 26, e-mail: books@springer.at, Internet: **www.springer.at**
D-69126 Heidelberg, Haberstraße 7, Fax +49.6221.345-229, e-mail: orders@springer.de
USA, Secaucus, NJ 07096-2485, P.O. Box 2485, Fax +1.201.348-4505, e-mail: orders@springer-ny.com
Eastern Book Service, Japan, Tokyo 113, 3–13, Hongo 3-chome, Bunkyo-ku, Fax +81.3.38 18 08 64, e-mail: orders@svt-ebs.co.jp

SpringerMedicine

Clemens Fritsch, Thomas Ruzicka

Fluorescence Diagnosis and Photodynamic Therapy of Skin Diseases

Atlas and Handbook

2003. Approx. 160 pages. Approx. 270 figures, in colour.
Hardcover **EUR 150,–**
(Recommended retail price)
Net-price subject to local VAT.
ISBN 3-211-83827-9
Due Spring 2003

This book is the most up-to-date publication on fluorescence diagnostic (FDAP) and photodynamic therapy (PDT) methods used in dermatology. Both techniques are presently world wide introduced as standards for the delineation and the treatment of cutaneous precancerous stages and tumors, which show steadily increasing numbers due to e.g. more frequent sun exposure.

Summarizing experiences on more than 5.000 treated patients, it offers a comprehensive information on every aspect of skin tumor detection and treatment. The main part of the book focuses on the clinical aspects giving detailed descriptions on skin tumor detection as well as photodynamic treatment of selected diseases (solar keratoses, basal cell carcinomas, squamous cell carcinomas, Bowen's disease, psoriasis lesions, etc.).

The clinically oriented chapters are supplemented by practical guidelines for PDT and FDAP. The included atlas is comprised of 270 high quality color figures allowing daily use as a handbook.

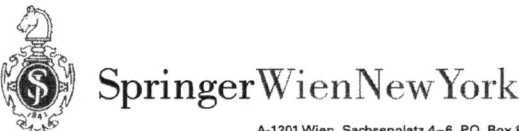

SpringerWienNewYork

A-1201 Wien, Sachsenplatz 4–6, P.O. Box 89, Fax +43.1.330 24 26, e-mail: books@springer.at, Internet: **www.springer.at**
D-69126 Heidelberg, Haberstraße 7, Fax +49.6221.345-229, e-mail: orders@springer.de
USA, Secaucus, NJ 07096-2485, P.O. Box 2485, Fax +1.201.348-4505, e-mail: orders@springer-ny.com
Eastern Book Service, Japan, Tokyo 113, 3–13, Hongo 3-chome, Bunkyo-ku, Fax +81.3.38 18 08 64, e-mail: orders@svt-ebs.co.jp

SpringerMedicine

Helmut Schenkel-Brunner

Human Blood Groups

Chemical and Biochemical
Basis of Antigen Specificity

Second, completely revised edition.
2000. XV, 637 pages. 173 figures.
Hardcover **EUR 106,–**
(Recommended retail price)
Net-price subject to local VAT.
ISBN 3-211-83471-0

This monograph covers the entire field of blood group serology, with its main emphasis on the chemical and biochemical basis of blood group specificity. Full consideration is given to molecular biology investigations, in particular to studies on the structure of blood group genes and the molecular biological basis of alleles and rare blood group variants, whereby relevant literature up to the year 2000 is covered.

The text is supplemented by numerous illustrations and tables, and detailed reference lists. The five years since the publication of the first edition have brought further advances in blood group research. Thanks to modern molecular biology, scientists have not only been able to identify the bearer molecules of many more blood groups, they have clarified the molecular basis of a number of further blood group specifities as well, offering a concise survey for use by blood bankers and researchers in biochemistry, blood group serology, immunohematology, forensic medicine, population genetics, and anthropology.

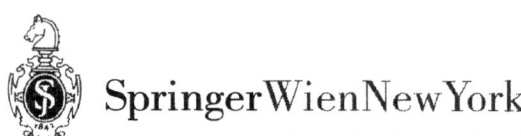

SpringerWienNewYork

A-1201 Wien, Sachsenplatz 4–6, P.O. Box 89, Fax +43.1.330 24 26, e-mail: books@springer.at, Internet: **www.springer.at**
D-69126 Heidelberg, Haberstraße 7, Fax +49.6221.345-229, e-mail: orders@springer.de
USA, Secaucus, NJ 07096-2485, P.O. Box 2485, Fax +1.201.348-4505, e-mail: orders@springer-ny.com
Eastern Book Service, Japan, Tokyo 113, 3–13, Hongo 3-chome, Bunkyo-ku, Fax +81.3.38 18 08 64, e-mail: orders@svt-ebs.co.jp

SpringerMedicine

P. Riederer, D. B. Calne, R. Horowski, Y. Mizuno, W. Poewe, M. Youdim (eds.)

Advances in Research on Neurodegeneration Volume 8

2000. VIII, 421 pages. 65 figures, partly in colour.

Hardcover **EUR 133,–**

(Recommended retail price) Net-price subject to local VAT.

(Special Edition of "Journal of Neural Transmission", Suppl. 60, 2000)

ISBN 3-211-83538-5

This volume highlightens recent advances in the research of neuro-degenerative processes and cell death. Also the role of inflammation in neurodegenerative processes is elucidated. A respectable number of articles deals with neuroprotective/neuroregenerative strategies. Although most of this work is preclinical, there is also first evidence from clinical studies that neuroprotection should be possible in neurodegenerative disorders like Parkinson's disease, amyotropic lateral sclerosis, Huntington's Chorea and eventually also Alzheimer's disease. Top scientists and international opinion leaders have discussed and lectured at the 8th International Winter Conference on Neurodegeneration (IWCN) in Tegernsee, Bavaria, Germany, from February 9–13, 2000. They have put together a valuable, comprehensive and timely piece of work that reviews all the above mentioned problems and tries to evaluate therapeutic strategies of the future.

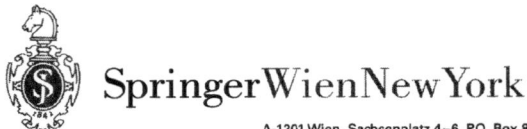

SpringerWienNewYork

A-1201 Wien, Sachsenplatz 4–6, P.O. Box 89, Fax +43.1.330 24 26, e-mail: books@springer.at, Internet: **www.springer.at**
D-69126 Heidelberg, Haberstraße 7, Fax +49.6221.345-229, e-mail: orders@springer.de
USA, Secaucus, NJ 07096-2485, P.O. Box 2485, Fax +1.201.348-4505, e-mail: orders@springer-ny.com
Eastern Book Service, Japan, Tokyo 113, 3–13, Hongo 3-chome, Bunkyo-ku, Fax +81.3.38 18 08 64, e-mail: orders@svt-ebs.co.jp

Springer-Verlag
and the Environment